SEPSIS WARRIOR

My Journey of Hope and Healing After Battling Sepsis 13 Times

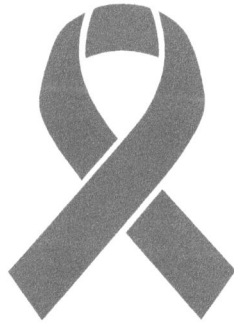

SANDRA KLEIER

Foreword By: Megan Jones, Director, Community Education and Support, Sepsis Alliance

Sandra Kleier-- 1ˢᵗ ed.
Chief Editor, Shannon Buritz
ISBN: 978-1-954757-65-3

The Publisher has strived to be as accurate and complete as possible in the creation of this book.

This book is not intended for use as a legal, business, accounting, or financial advice source. All readers are advised to seek the services of competent professionals in legal, business, accounting, and finance fields.

Like anything else in life, there are no guarantees of income or results in practical advice books. Readers are cautioned to rely on their judgment about their individual circumstances to act accordingly.

While all attempts have been made to verify information provided in this publication, the Publisher assumes no responsibility for errors, omissions, or contrary interpretation of the subject matter herein. Any perceived slights of specific persons, peoples, or organizations are unintentional.

I dedicate this book to my husband, Ron, who has stood faithfully by my side through every trial. Since my first brush with death twelve years ago, he has selflessly taken on the role of caregiver, becoming my nurse around the clock. His unwavering love and encouragement have carried me through each step of my sepsis journey.

I also dedicate this to my daughters, who walk beside me day in and day out, and who help Ron advocate for me when I can't speak for myself, and to my other children, whose love and prayers surround me always.

To my dearest friend since grade school, who has listened with compassion on both my best and worst days. And to my lifelong classmates, whose steady support for me and my family has never wavered during each hospital stay, I am forever grateful.

To Megan at Sepsis Alliance, who has encouraged my advocacy and become a valuable friend. To my sepsis brothers and sisters, who I've met through Sepsis Alliance, who have uplifted me along my journey in ways that they'll never know.

To sepsis survivors everywhere: I dedicate this book to you with the hope that you know your life, though forever changed by sepsis, still holds immense value. You remain an important part of society, and no matter your circumstances, you can continue to live a long, meaningful, and fulfilling life.

CONTENTS

FOREWORD

I first met Sandra Kleier almost four years ago, when I had just come to work at Sepsis Alliance and was beginning to develop the virtual support community which would become Sepsis Alliance Connect. Sandra was one of the first people to raise her hand to help us identify what sepsis survivors like her might need, but I quickly learned something much more valuable: how much sepsis survivors like Sandra have to offer.

While medical professionals with a long list of credentials after their name may be the experts on the medical process of sepsis, survivors like Sandra are the experts regarding what comes next: the experience of moving forward, changed. They are the ones who know best what to say to the people finding themselves on that same challenging path, giving advice on how to make it through the tough days while celebrating the good ones.

In my privileged position, getting to know survivors like Sandra (and the others whose stories are included in the following pages), I've been lucky enough to witness the wisdom that comes from persevering through adversity. I've been a fly on the wall as compassion has been offered in someone's darkest moments, and later laughed myself to tears at the absurdly hilarious stories that can only be shared between those who truly "get it." I count myself truly lucky to be an observer of these conversations.

If you're a recent sepsis survivor, I hope this book provides you a link to "your people," and perhaps a first step toward connecting with others who have been where you are now. If you are supporting a loved one, I trust that what follows will serve as a window into the things they may struggle to share with you. And if you're someone whose connection to sepsis is a professional one, perhaps you might find in these pages a resource- not just in what is printed here, but in the experiences of those people like Sandra, who have earned their expertise in what comes after sepsis, step by sometimes excruciating step.

Gratefully,

Megan Jones
Director, Community Education and Support
Sepsis Alliance

INTRODUCTION

For us sepsis survivors, the road to recovery isn't just about healing wounds; it's about discovering a new sense of self-worth and finding a renewed purpose in life. It's a journey of personal growth and transformation. I have become more empathetic and compassionate towards others as I navigate the physical and mental challenges. I even feel like I've been given a second chance at life. This becomes a driving force for positive change, not just in my own life but in the lives of those around me. It's a pull towards something bigger, a calling to raise awareness and advocate for others going through what I did. My goal is to help shape a future where sepsis is better understood, where survivors are better supported, and where no one has to feel alone.

Breaking Down Barriers

Surviving sepsis is a significant achievement, but the road doesn't end there. I have felt a complex mix of physical and emotional struggles that come with the road to recovery. These challenges can be overwhelming, and I often feel like I am fighting a battle on multiple fronts, even to this day.

One of the biggest barriers is the emotional toll that sepsis takes. Survivors often face post-traumatic stress disorder (PTSD) and post-sepsis syndrome (PSS), which can manifest as depression, loneliness, and a sense of isolation. These feelings are compounded by a sense of not being understood or having their experiences minimized by others, especially because there is a lack of information about post-sepsis syndrome in the medical community. PSS can bring overwhelming fatigue, cognitive deficits, muscle pain, nightmares, and difficulty walking and performing everyday tasks. These symptoms make even the simplest tasks seem monumental, exacerbating feelings of helplessness and frustration.

I would go to the doctor, hoping for answers, and they might do some tests, but when those tests came back normal, it was incredibly frustrating to feel like you knew something was wrong with your body that couldn't be validated. I started questioning myself, wondering if it was just in my head. But deep down, I knew I wasn't crazy. Part of the problem is that post-sepsis syndrome is a relatively new diagnosis in the medical community, so doctors are not equipped to diagnose or treat it.

There is some good news, though. With the emergence of COVID-19 and long COVID, there's been a growing awareness of these types of post-illness syndromes. Long COVID shares many of the same symptoms as post-sepsis syndrome—fatigue, muscle aches, cognitive deficits, malaise—*and* they both involve cytokine storms. This excessive immune response causes inflammation and damage in the body. This similarity has brought more attention to post-sepsis syndrome; in fact, now there's an ICD-10 code for it, which means it's officially recognized as a medical condition. With this recognition, doctors are learning more about it, which is a huge step forward. As the medical community becomes more aware of post-sepsis syndrome, you'll have more doctors who understand what you're going through. It's a process, but we're moving in the right direction.

Support and understanding are crucial for breaking down these barriers. Survivors need effective coping mechanisms to be successful on the road to recovery. I recently heard from a young lady who had just been out of the hospital for a week. She felt like she was going crazy—her thoughts were bouncing around in her head, and she feared she was experiencing cognitive decline or even a mental breakdown. Fortunately, she found a support group just in time. After talking to others who had been through similar experiences, she felt a sense of relief and hope. It was a turning point for her, and she began believing she could make it through. Stories like this are what make this mission worth it to me.

Facing Your Fears and Suspicions

When you've survived sepsis, it's only natural to have fears about the future. I hear from survivors all the time, "Am I going to get sepsis again?" and "What if this is as good as it gets?"

Let's start with the first fear: Will I get sepsis again?

Unfortunately, survivors have about a 50% higher chance of becoming septic within the first two years compared to the general population. That's a sobering statistic, but it doesn't mean you're helpless. The key is education. You need to know the signs and symptoms of sepsis and quickly act if they appear. If you start running a fever, don't wait to see if it goes away. Go straight to the emergency room. Not urgent care, not your doctor's office—the ER. And make sure you tell them you've had sepsis before. The sooner you get help, the less severe and traumatic it will be. At the very least, ask them to do blood cultures and general lab work, i.e., CBC, CMP, lactic acid, etc. There's no shame in going to the emergency room and being sent home!

The second fear—what if this is as good as it gets?—is a little more complex. It's easy to feel trapped in the idea that your best days are behind you, that your body will never be the same, or that you'll never regain your strength, but that's where a shift in mindset can make all the difference. Start by focusing on the good in your life. Instead of dwelling on what you can't do, think about what you can. Set small daily goals, even just one or two things. It could be as simple as taking a short walk or returning an email. At the end of each day, list something you're thankful for. It doesn't have to be big—sometimes, the little things mean the most. I found much to be grateful for as I looked for the positive. I learned that time is precious and didn't want to waste it on negative thoughts or regrets. I wanted to make the most of every moment to the best of my capabilities.

You might have questions and suspicions about how you got

sepsis. The need to find a reason or a cause is a normal part of coping. Two suspicions I hear a lot are, "Did I pick up sepsis in the hospital?" and "Did the doctor make a mistake?"

First, let's address the suspicion about picking up sepsis in the hospital. Sepsis isn't a bacteria or a virus; it's the body's immune response to an infection already there. The infection can come from many sources—a bug bite, a scratch, a common cold that turns into pneumonia, or something else entirely. So, while some people pick up infections in the hospital, like from a nurse or doctor who doesn't wash their hands, most people had the infection before they arrived.

That leads to a second suspicion: Did the doctor make a mistake? This one usually comes up after a surgery or medical procedure. People think, "Did the doctor nick something?" or "Did they mess up and just not tell me?" Infection and even "nicks" can indeed be a complication of surgery, and it's usually listed in the pre-op consent form you sign before the procedure. But that doesn't mean the doctor caused it. It's a risk that's part of the surgery and can happen without any error or negligence from the medical team. The reality is that most doctors are doing their best, and sepsis can occur despite all the proper precautions.

If you're feeling suspicious or unsure about how you got sepsis, it's okay to ask questions and seek clarification. Get a copy of your medical records, talk to your doctors about interpreting the reports, find support groups, and get informed. The more you know, the more you can focus on your recovery and let go of the doubts holding you back. Sepsis can happen to anyone, and it's not always straightforward. But with the right knowledge and support, you can confidently move forward.

Throughout the pages of this book, I hope to give you that confidence by providing answers to these common questions:

- *"How did I get sepsis?"*
- *"Will I ever recover physically or mentally and get back to normal?"*
- *"Will I get sepsis again?"*

And more...

Defining Success

Finding peace within myself and the ability to move forward with my life was my definition of success. After enduring such a traumatic experience, achieving that sense of inner calm was a huge step. It signaled that I had come to terms with what happened and was ready to share my story.

Success can manifest in different ways. It might be gaining the confidence to talk about your experience with friends and family. It takes courage to open up about something so personal, especially when sepsis is often misunderstood. But when you do, you're not just healing yourself; you're educating those around you about sepsis and how it affects people.

For some survivors, success means taking their story beyond their close circle. Maybe it's volunteering at the hospital where they were treated, giving thanks to the staff who helped save their life. It could be as simple as writing a thank-you note or bringing a small gift as a token of appreciation. These small acts of gratitude can be incredibly meaningful for you and the medical professionals who played a part in your recovery.

Another way to measure success is by becoming an advocate for sepsis awareness, which is a powerful thing to be. Some survivors find fulfillment in speaking to nursing classes or community groups, sharing their stories to help others understand what sepsis is and how to respond if someone they know is affected.

You might wonder why I'm the person to guide you on your mission to a successful sepsis recovery. I'm a 12-time sepsis survivor. My story didn't start with a sepsis diagnosis—it began years before with digestive problems and bowel obstructions that led me to the hospital for emergency surgery. The pain was unbearable, and I just wanted relief. But when I woke up on a ventilator, unable to move, I knew that my life had changed.

The first bout of sepsis was intense, with fatigue like I'd never felt before. After eight days in the hospital and a second surgery six months later, it took about a year before I finally started to feel like I might live again. But it was just the beginning. Two years later, since I could no longer eat solid food, I needed to start Total Parenteral Nutrition or TPN. This unique sterile intravenous (IV) solution is given directly into the bloodstream via a portacath inserted into the internal jugular vein, which terminates in the superior vena cava. The portacath and the high sugar content in the TPN formula make for a high risk of infection. The doctors told me, "It's not a matter of if you'll get sepsis, it's when." And they were right—I was back in the ER within 30 days with a high fever and rigors, rapid temperature rise, violent, uncontrollable shaking, teeth chattering so hard I thought my teeth would break, and feeling extremely cold even when my body was warming up.

Since then, I've faced sepsis 12 times, septic shock twice, and been on a ventilator once. My most recent sepsis episode was in January 2022—a fungal infection, which is as serious as it gets. Thankfully, I've been on prophylactic antibiotics since then, and I've managed to stay out of the hospital.

Through all of this, I've experienced every emotion possible—depression, anger, bargaining, and, eventually, acceptance. The early days were dark, and I did not know if I could walk or handle activities of daily living. I spent years just existing, surviving, and wondering if this was my life from now on. I'd been an RN since 1991. Nursing and taking care of others were all I knew. It remains a daily struggle as I still suffer from many comorbidities that have reared their ugly heads from damage left behind to organs and body structures thanks to sepsis.

But despite the very real daily struggles, something had shifted. I decided that this wasn't who I wanted to be, and I wasn't going to let sepsis define me. I found my way to acceptance, asking myself, "What will I do with the rest of my life so that I feel valuable?"

I decided to write this book because, after reading so many books about sepsis, I realized that most of them focus on one person's unique story, diving deep into their specific experiences with ICU sedation and psychosis. While those stories are valid, I feel they often miss the broader picture—what most sepsis survivors actually go through. My goal is to speak to the common struggles we face: memory fog, overwhelming fatigue, and the loss of the ability to do everyday activities. These challenges are exhausting and, frankly, not often talked about.

I also wanted to provide a resource for sepsis survivors who feel isolated as they navigate recovery, not knowing that there's a whole community of survivors and advocates who understand what they're going through. I couldn't find a book offering this kind of guidance, so I created it myself.

Remember, you've already shown incredible strength by surviving sepsis. Now, you have the opportunity to reclaim your life, find your purpose, and even become an advocate for others. Together, we can raise awareness about sepsis, improve understanding in the medical community, and ensure that no one has to face this journey alone.

- Sandra Kleier

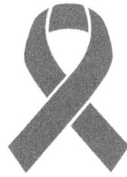

CHAPTER ONE
UNDERSTANDING SEPSIS

This chapter is designed to educate you about sepsis and how to recognize its symptoms. Understanding this information can be lifesaving, as sepsis is a medical emergency that demands immediate attention.

Sepsis is your body's extreme reaction to an infection. Typically, your immune system fights infections, but sometimes it can overreact, leading to widespread inflammation. This inflammation can damage normal tissues and organs, leading to organ failure and even death. It's a life-threatening condition that can escalate quickly if not treated urgently.

Sepsis can arise from various types of infections:

- **Bacterial Infections:** The most common causes include kidney stones, urinary tract infections, pneumonia, peritonitis from an abdominal perforation, and infections from lacerations, bug bites, or implantable devices.

- **Viral Infections**: Viruses like influenza (the flu) or COVID-19 can lead to sepsis.
- **Fungal Infections**: Infections caused by yeast or molds.
- **Non-Infectious Insults**: Trauma from injuries like car accidents can also trigger sepsis. Sometimes, the exact cause remains unidentified, which can be particularly frustrating.

I've experienced sepsis twelve times. My first sepsis episode was due to peritonitis from a small bowel perforation. Subsequent infections were related to complications with an implantable port in my chest, including bacterial and fungal infections. The 11th incident involved a urinary tract infection that migrated to my port; the 12th was a fungal infection in the same port.

One of the most frightening moments was in pre-op, before my bowel perforation surgery, when they couldn't get a blood pressure reading on me. It wasn't until I saw my daughter, who is a nurse, crying with the pre-op nurses that I understood the seriousness of the situation. I overheard a nurse telling the doctor that my lactic acid level was 7.5, which is extremely high. I was in severe pain from pancreatitis and my perforated bowel, and I was desperate for this pain to end. I remember asking the doctor if I was going to die. Although I don't recall his complete response, he assured me the safest place for me was in the operating room.

Another bout of sepsis in July of 2021 led to persistent back pain by September. My nursing background told me I should have improved with rest, NSAIDs (nonsteroidal anti-inflammatory drugs), and gentle stretching after about six weeks. However, the pain only worsened, and by November, it became unbearable. Reluctant to visit the emergency room, I went to urgent care for X-rays. The radiologist immediately advised me to go to the ER. I was diagnosed with osteomyelitis (bone infection), discitis (infection in the discs between the vertebrae), and burst fractures of the T9 and T10 vertebrae, compressing my spinal cord. Although this wasn't another instance of sepsis, it was directly related to my previous infection.

Understanding sepsis and recognizing its symptoms can truly be a matter of life and death. My personal experiences highlight how quickly sepsis can escalate and how its effects can linger long after the immediate threat has passed. By sharing this, I hope to emphasize the importance of prompt medical attention and ongoing vigilance, especially for those at higher risk. Being informed and proactive can make all the difference in managing and surviving sepsis.

Changing Perceptions of Sepsis

Before my diagnosis, my understanding of sepsis was quite limited. My nursing program, which I attended in the early 90s, didn't focus much on sepsis. It was more commonly referred to as "blood poisoning" by the layperson. I reached out to some of my classmates, and they had similar recollections—sepsis wasn't a topic we covered in depth.

I recall my first encounter with a sepsis patient, though I didn't know at the time that was what he had. As a new graduate nurse in 1991, I had a patient fresh out of surgery. He showed troubling signs—no urine output all night, low blood pressure, and he didn't wake up at all. He didn't have a fever, and his heart rate and oxygen saturation were normal. The lack of urine output and low blood pressure were especially concerning, so I urged my night nurse supervisor to check on him. Finally, after midnight, we assessed him together, and we admitted him to the ICU. He pulled through, but it was a lesson I never forgot.

Back then, I thought most people died from sepsis, and that was probably true in many cases. I couldn't find specific statistics from that time, but it wasn't until I was recovering and researching online that I learned more about the survival rates and long-term impacts.

My perception of sepsis changed dramatically after becoming directly affected by it. I realized that many people do survive sepsis, but at least 50% of survivors continue to experience symptoms and lifelong effects. That realization was frightening. Initially, I believed I was strong and resilient, thinking I wouldn't be affected in the long term. I expected to recover and regain my strength. But as the months passed and I reached the one-year mark without returning to "normal," I became depressed. Accepting that I might be among those who wouldn't fully recover was a harsh reality.

At that time, there weren't many resources available for sepsis survivors. Close to my one year anniversary, I sought counseling to help me cope with the significant changes in my life and the emotions that came with them, which I highly recommend to others in similar scenarios.

Coming to Terms with Sepsis

When I first discovered I had experienced septic shock, it was a shock in itself. I didn't hear about it from the doctors at the hospital; instead, I found out from my dictated discharge summary a week after I was sent home. It was a surreal moment. The hospital staff didn't bring it up, and I think part of the reason is that discussing sepsis isn't common practice. Even though I had some knowledge about sepsis, my cognitive function was so impaired that it didn't register that this was what I was experiencing.

Seeing those words in my discharge summary hit me hard. It was a reality check—realizing that I had come so close to death. The grief began. It made sense why I was so upset, and why simple tasks like getting cleaned up every day were so exhausting. It made sense as to why I was so moody and forgetful.

Initially, I believed there would be a straightforward recovery period, after which I'd return to my usual self. My surgeon mentioned that it might take about six months for me to feel better, especially since I had another surgery planned. But as

I started researching sepsis and its aftermath, I realized that while some people do return to their baseline, many do not. At that point, I was naive, thinking I would bounce back by the end. Little did I know how much my life and health would change.

Like many others, I thought I would be fully healed once I completed my antibiotics. However, experiencing sepsis first-hand shattered this misconception. I learned that at least 50% of survivors suffer from Post-Sepsis Syndrome (PSS), which includes a range of lingering symptoms like cognitive deficiencies (memory loss and brain fog), chronic fatigue, sleep disturbances (mainly insomnia, though some people sleep excessively), muscle or joint pain, hair loss, depression, anxiety, PTSD, and nightmares. These symptoms can persist for months or even years.

Understanding PSS and realizing that these symptoms could be a long-term reality made me feel like I was losing my mind, thinking this was how life would be forever. I went through the Kübler-Ross stages of grief: denial, anger, bargaining, depression, and acceptance.

- **Denial**: Initially, I couldn't accept what I had gone through. I knew I had nearly died, but part of me denied the severity of my experience, downplaying it.
- **Anger**: I was angry. I had a strong personal identity all of my life. Why couldn't I overcome this frail persona? And why had the doctors waited so long to treat me?

- **Bargaining**: I found myself making promises, hoping for a return to some semblance of my old self. "If I can just get back to normal, I promise to help others and volunteer more."
- **Depression**: This stage was particularly tough. Coming to terms with the realization that my life had changed irrevocably and fearing it would never improve was overwhelming. At this point, I knew I'd probably never be able to work as an RN again.
- **Acceptance**: Finally, I reached a point of acceptance. I acknowledged what had happened and started rebuilding my life, learning from my experiences and considering how to use them to help others.

This journey through the stages of grief was challenging but necessary. It allowed me to confront my new reality and find a way to move forward, turning my experience into a source of strength and purpose.

Family and Friends' Reactions

When my family learned about my diagnosis, their reactions varied. My daughter and stepdaughter, both registered nurses, understood the gravity of the situation. My other daughters, my husband Ron and my mother, Betty, were more generally upset, not grasping the severity of what had happened. Ron, who became my primary caregiver, had to adapt quickly, essentially becoming a nurse overnight, and he did an excellent job.

The rest of my family and friends, including the grandkids and neighbors, knew I had been seriously ill and needed rest, but they didn't understand the full extent of it. My mother frequently asked about the cause, wondering if it was hereditary. During my recovery, I did extensive research, mostly while bedridden, but I often kept what I learned to myself. However, I could talk openly with my daughters, who helped me piece together the sequence of events and share our feelings about what we had all been through. My best friend since grade school, who now lives in South Carolina, probably lost her hearing listening to me all of these years.

Even now, my husband doesn't like to discuss that time. He's incredibly supportive of my healing and my work moving forward, but he doesn't engage much in conversations about his emotions from that period. Many of my friends still don't understand the ongoing impact of sepsis. They often assume that because I'm not visibly ill anymore, I must be fully recovered, which isn't the case. It requires a lot of education to help people understand the lasting effects.

Public and Medical Community Understanding of Sepsis

I believe sepsis needs to be better understood by the public and the medical community. When I discuss post-sepsis syndrome and its related comorbidities with most of my doctors, they tend to gloss over the subject. My primary care physician,

Dr. Newkirk, is the exception. He listens and works with me to brainstorm potential solutions, which makes me feel heard and validated, even if we don't always find definitive answers.

This lack of acknowledgment from other medical professionals is disheartening. For example, my nephrologist won't discuss whether my chronic kidney issues are due to the strong antibiotics and vasopressors used during my treatment or the lack of oxygen when I had a sepsis infection. It isn't easy to move forward when doctors don't validate your feelings or acknowledge post-sepsis syndrome. It feels like a constant struggle to be taken seriously, which can be emotionally draining.

As for the general public, it's challenging for people to understand or identify with sepsis if they have yet to experience it or learn much about it. I hope that by sharing my story, people might remember it if they ever find themselves or a loved one getting rapidly worse. It could make a crucial difference in recognizing the symptoms of sepsis in time to save lives.

A New Perspective on Health and Life

My journey with sepsis has profoundly reshaped how I view health and life. I've learned not to take any day for granted and to focus more on the present rather than worrying about the future. Change starts from within, and while I now face many physical limitations, my mind remains active and capable. I write notes to remind myself of tasks, checking them off as I complete them. This simple practice helps me stay organized and provides a sense of accomplishment.

Another significant part of my healing journey is facilitating a support group for sepsis survivors via Zoom. This group has been invaluable. It allows us to connect with others who truly understand what we're going through, validating our experiences and feelings. Through these conversations, we've come to believe that, in a way, sepsis has made us better people. We share a sense of gratitude for this renewed appreciation of life that perhaps we wouldn't have gained otherwise.

Sepsis is a challenging journey that doesn't end with hospital discharge. It's a continuous process of adaptation and finding new ways to live fully. Sharing our stories and supporting each other can help educate and empower more people to recognize the signs of sepsis and advocate for their health. Finding strength in shared experiences provides hope for a better future.

KEY TAKEAWAYS

➤ Sepsis is a life-threatening condition that requires immediate medical attention due to its rapid progression and potential to cause organ failure and death.

➤ It can result from various infections, including bacterial, viral, fungal, and even non-infectious causes. Awareness of sepsis symptoms and their urgency is crucial for timely intervention.

➤ Personal experiences, like my repeated battles with sepsis, highlight the severity and lasting impact of the condition, including Post-Sepsis Syndrome, which affects many survivors with chronic symptoms.

➤ The medical community and public often lack sufficient understanding and recognition of sepsis and its long-term effects, making advocacy and education vital.

➤ A supportive community and open discussion about sepsis can help survivors navigate their recovery and cope with the emotional and physical challenges of the syndrome.

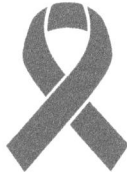

CHAPTER TWO

STAGES OF SEPSIS

Being able to recognize the stages of sepsis can save your life. Knowing what signs and symptoms to watch for means you can seek help before it escalates into an emergency. It isn't a single-step progression; it moves through identifiable stages, each with increasing severity.

Sepsis

Sepsis begins when the body shows signs of infection but has started reacting in ways that can damage its own tissues and organs. You may notice:

- **Fever:** A temperature higher than 100.4°F or lower than 96.8°F.
- **Respiratory Rate:** Breathing becomes rapid, more than 20 breaths per minute.

- **Heart Rate:** A pulse rate above 90 beats per minute.
- **White Blood Cell Count:** Increased WBC count over 12,000 or below 4,000, with over 10% immature cells (bands).
- **PCO$_2$ Levels:** Below 32 mmHg.

In this stage, symptoms may include chills, teeth chattering, extreme fatigue, and the beginnings of shortness of breath and cognitive decline.

Severe Sepsis

If sepsis isn't controlled, it progresses into severe sepsis, where organs begin to struggle. Here's what that looks like:

- **Signs of Organ Dysfunction:** Issues like trouble breathing as the lungs become compromised, drastically low or no urine output indicating kidney stress, abnormal liver test results, and changes in mental status.
- **Hypotension:** A sudden drop in blood pressure (systolic BP under 90).
- **Lactate Levels:** A lactate reading above 4 mmol shows that the body isn't getting enough oxygen to the tissues.

This stage of sepsis is frightening because the body is struggling more visibly, and symptoms become severe. Breathing feels labored, and there's a heavy fatigue that's overwhelming.

Septic Shock

Septic shock is the most severe stage, and by now, the body is in a life-threatening crisis.

- **Persisting Signs of Organ Damage:** The organs begin to fail without proper intervention.
- **Critically Low Blood Pressure:** Blood pressure remains dangerously low (systolic BP under 90), even with fluids.
- **High Lactate Levels:** Persistent lactate levels above 4 mmol.

At this stage, the blood pressure drops to life-threatening levels, and the organs can't function properly. This is an emergency, and every second counts in getting medical help.

In the following sections, we'll go into the details of each stage based on my personal experience. Sepsis has tried to take me down twelve times, but by recognizing these stages, I've fought back every time. I want to share what I learned so you can have the knowledge and strength to respond to sepsis in its earliest stages.

What Are the
Three Stages of Sepsis?

Stage 1: Sepsis

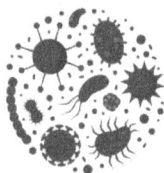

Sepsis begins when the body shows signs of infection but has started reacting in ways that can damage its own tissues and organs. You may notice:

Fever: A temperature higher than 100.4°F or lower than 96.8°F.

Respiratory Rate: Breathing becomes rapid, more than 20 breaths per minute.

Heart Rate: A pulse rate above 90 beats per minute.

White Blood Cell Count: Increased WBC count over 12,000 or below 4,000, with over 10% immature cells (bands).

PCO^2 Levels: Below 32 mmHg.

In this stage, symptoms may include chills, teeth chattering, extreme fatigue, and the beginnings of shortness of breath and cognitive decline.

Stage 2: Severe Sepsis

If sepsis isn't controlled, it progresses into severe sepsis, where organs begin to struggle.
Here's what that looks like:

Signs of Organ Dysfunction: Issues like trouble breathing as the lungs become compromised, drastically low or no urine output indicating kidney stress, abnormal liver test results, and changes in mental status.

Hypotension: A sudden drop in blood pressure (systolic BP under 90).

Lactate Levels: A lactate reading above 4 mmol shows that the body isn't getting enough oxygen to the tissues.

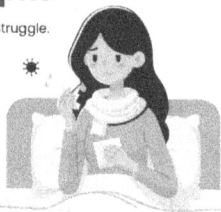

This stage of sepsis is frightening because the body is struggling more visibly, and symptoms become severe. Breathing feels labored, and there's a heavy fatigue that's overwhelming.

Stage 3: Sepsis Shock

Septic shock is the most severe stage, and by now, the body is in a life-threatening crisis.

Persisting Signs of Organ Damage: The organs begin to fail without proper intervention.

Critically Low Blood Pressure: Blood pressure remains dangerously low (systolic BP under 90), even with fluids.

High Lactate Levels: Persistent lactate levels above 4 mmol.

At this stage, the blood pressure drops to life-threatening levels, and the organs can't function properly. This is an emergency, and every second counts in getting medical help.

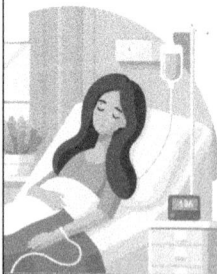

The First Signs: Knowing When Something's Really Wrong

The first time sepsis invaded my life, it felt nothing like what I expected. It all started with something as simple as a cheeseburger for lunch. I'd felt perfectly fine until I started feeling nauseous, with a dull ache in my stomach. At first, I thought, "Maybe I'm just coming down with a stomach bug." The pain started building slowly but steadily, becoming a deep, rolling ache that came in waves. When I got home, I could tell this was more than an upset stomach. I had to lie down. Something wasn't right.

By early evening, my nausea turned into dry heaves. Every fifteen minutes, another wave hit, but unlike normal vomiting, there was no relief afterward. It was just empty, painful heaving, and it was taking every ounce of strength I had left. The pain kept getting sharper, digging into my gut and spreading. Soon, I was in so much pain that even the slightest movement felt unbearable. I couldn't make it to the car; we had no choice but to call an ambulance.

I remember every second of that ride, and let me tell you, the experience was nothing like the emergency scenes on TV. No rushing lights or sirens were blaring; the ride was painfully s-l-o-w, every bump jarring my body. On top of that, the head paramedic was smugly indifferent. He wouldn't even help me get onto the gurney, insisting I just had the flu. I was left to crawl, inch-by-inch, over to the stretcher and pull myself up onto it, screaming in pain all the while. The cold metal of the ambulance cot made it feel like my body was freezing from the outside while it burned up on the inside.

When I experienced my second major infection two years after the bowel perforation, I knew more about sepsis than I ever wanted to. I'd read everything I could about the signs, symptoms, and what to watch for, and thank goodness I did. When the chills hit, it was like a freight train. Within ten minutes, I went from feeling just a little cold to uncontrollable shivering, my teeth chattering so violently I thought they might crack. I'd check my temperature, and without fail, it would be a manageable 99.9°F. But I quickly trusted my intuition that if I didn't act fast, it would soon spike to 102 or 103°F, sometimes within another fifteen minutes. I started keeping a bag packed, ready to rush out the door.

With one of my later infections, the symptoms were terrifyingly visual. I was hooking up my TPN (the IV nutrition I rely on) to my port, just like I did every day, but this time, something was wrong. Almost instantly, I saw redness spreading across the vein in my chest, like a line creeping up toward my neck. In minutes, my whole breast was red and burning hot to the touch. I didn't need any more signs; we rushed to the ER.

Each time, the symptoms came on quickly and escalated even faster. I couldn't afford to waste time wondering if this was "just a fever." By then, I had learned to respect the speed and severity of sepsis. I kept my bags packed and my husband on alert, and we knew the drill: the second a fever hit, we were out the door. Sepsis doesn't wait, and neither could I.

S	**E**	**P**	**S**	**I**	**S**
Shivering, fever, or very cold	**E**xtreme pain or general discomfort ("worst ever")	**P**ale or discolored skin	**S**leepy, difficult to wake up, confused	"**I** feel like I might die"	**S**hort of breath

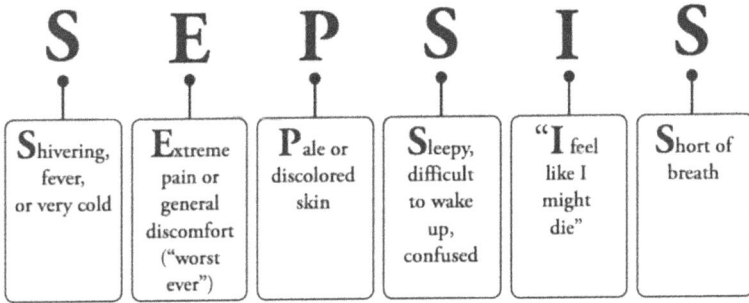

Image courtesy of: Sepsis Alliance

What I Wish I Had Known About Sepsis Early On

If there's one lesson I've learned repeatedly, timing is everything regarding sepsis. Looking back, I wish I'd known just how vital those first few signs really are. The sooner treatment starts, the less severe sepsis becomes, and that can make all the difference between life and death. The goal is to receive antibiotic therapy within an hour of arriving at the emergency room.

One thing I can't emphasize enough: do not take fever reducers. I know it's tempting to pop something to take the edge off but doing so can hide the symptoms you need to pay attention to. When sepsis starts, it often begins with chilling, a mild fever, a shift in mental clarity, or pain that doesn't feel normal. Don't wait to see if it goes away, or call your doctor for their opinion first. Take the signs seriously and head to the ER.

It's also important to educate your family. They need to know what to watch for, too, because sepsis can impact your mental state quickly, clouding your ability to recognize the danger. Signs like sudden chills, a shift in mental clarity, and unusual pain are all red flags.

Another very important suggestion is to tell the ER nurses and doctors that you have been septic in the past and wonder if it could be sepsis again.

When it comes to sepsis, remember
IT'S ABOUT TIME™. Watch for:

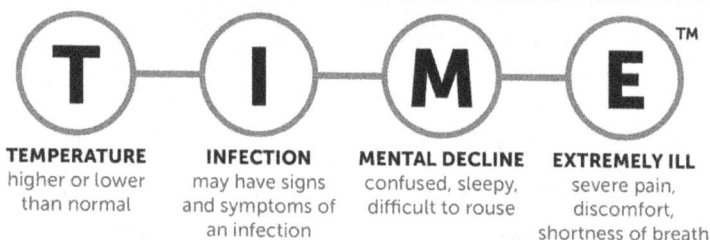

T	I	M	E™
TEMPERATURE higher or lower than normal	**INFECTION** may have signs and symptoms of an infection	**MENTAL DECLINE** confused, sleepy, difficult to rouse	**EXTREMELY ILL** severe pain, discomfort, shortness of breath

If you experience a combination of these symptoms: seek urgent medical care, call 911, or go to the hospital with an advocate. Ask: **"Could it be sepsis?"**

Image courtesy of: Sepsis Alliance

Crossing the Line: From First Signs to Severe Sepsis

The first time I transitioned from those early symptoms to something much more severe, it was like crossing an invisible line—one minute, I felt like myself, and the next, I was somewhere else entirely. I remember it felt like I was the only person in the universe. Even though my family and nurses surrounded me, they became part of the background.

I couldn't focus on them and didn't even feel fully aware of their presence. My mind was closed off like I only existed inside myself. I lacked the mental clarity even to comprehend how dire things had become. To the medical professionals reading this, please trust your instincts. Don't rely on a patient's perspective alone, especially when they're experiencing cognitive decline. At that point, I wasn't capable of assessing my own state.

The turning point came when a surgeon I knew well entered my room. His familiar face and touch brought me back to reality, even if only slightly. When he pressed down on my abdomen, I felt the rigidity, and that's when I understood—this was life-threatening. My mind couldn't fully grasp the details, but I recognized something was very wrong.

Once the surgeon confirmed the severity of my condition, everything kicked into high gear. The nurses started working rapidly, prepping me for surgery. I remember them inserting a second IV, setting up a Hibiclens bath to reduce infection risk, and taking me down to pre-op. At that stage, I couldn't process all the steps or details, but I could feel the urgency in their movements and the silent communication among the team. Their actions, though a blur to me then, saved my life.

Even when they could not palpate a blood pressure, or another nurse called out my current lactic acid lab value of 7.4 mmol, they didn't wait or hesitate—they acted calmly and purposefully. Even then, as I lay there in intractable pain, I was unaware of the storm raging in my body.

A Call for Change

One of the most frustrating aspects of my sepsis journey has been the lingering gaps in medical understanding and care. Despite all the advancements in identifying sepsis, it still feels like healthcare providers often miss the bigger picture—that sepsis doesn't end when a patient leaves the hospital. Recovery is a long, winding road, and Post-Sepsis Syndrome is a constant companion. When I go to the ER and tell them I've had sepsis twelve times, with two episodes progressing to septic shock, they take it seriously and immediately start checking vital signs, drawing blood, and doing physical assessments. I hear stories from other survivors all of the time that they went to the emergency room and weren't taken seriously or would be made to feel like they're just attention seekers needing some attention, or worse yet, drug seekers, and are sent home without even any blood work done. It's astonishing to me that patients still encounter disbelief or even dismissal. I always felt incredibly lucky to have my doctors at my hospital who always take me seriously. Then, it happened to me.

One night, I arrived at the ER with a fever of 102°F, my bags packed because I knew how this would likely end. My husband was out of town, my daughters were unavailable, and I had to make sure my dogs were cared for by my grandson. Yet, when I arrived, the fever had broken.

The medical team thought it was curious that I had brought my luggage, implying I was expecting to stay without cause.

They had only checked my blood pressure, and in the absence of a current temperature, they were going to send me home. I was exhausted, alone, and needing care, not judgment. I asked them for basic tests—blood cultures, simple blood work—and while they agreed, I felt humiliated by their lack of empathy. The doctor didn't even examine me. The experience was dehumanizing.

Unfortunately, these dismissive attitudes aren't isolated. Many doctors shrug off our concerns about long-term symptoms or sidestep conversations about the toll that powerful antibiotics and other treatments have taken on our kidneys. Each of these interactions is a painful reminder that the medical community still has a long way to go in understanding the full impact of sepsis on a survivor's life.

Thankfully, there are signs of change. A new ICD-10 code for post-sepsis care, **Z51.A,** may help providers take lingering effects seriously. Through Sepsis Alliance, I'm training with a group that educates healthcare professionals about recognizing sepsis and its aftermath. I'm both a registered nurse and a sepsis survivor, so I understand the clinical side as well as the emotional toll. We reach out to hospital and clinic staff to help them recognize sepsis's complex effects on patients. Every story I share and every session we lead is a step toward building a healthcare community that treats sepsis survivors with the dignity and understanding they deserve.

Recovery Reflections

Reflecting on my initial recovery process, I can say without a doubt that it was an eye-opening experience, and not always in ways I expected. I had been through major abdominal surgeries before, but this time was different. The fatigue was beyond anything I imagined—mind-numbing exhaustion that made even the smallest movements feel like climbing a mountain. I had a long incision from my sternum down to my pubic bone, and I needed a hospital bed just to get in and out of bed. The weakness took over everything. It would take me hours just to clean up for the day.

And then there was the brain fog. I've always been sharp with words; English was my strength. I even had a college professor—a tough-as-nails cat lady with a flair for making life difficult—who didn't believe in handing out A's. I'd survived her challenges, but this brain fog was something else entirely. It left me confused, struggling to find words, and feeling like a part of my identity had slipped away.

The pain was unrelenting, a constant ache that took over my body. I already had fibromyalgia, but after this surgery, the muscle and joint pain became so much worse. I couldn't get comfortable, couldn't find relief. All I wanted to do was sleep, but even that felt like a battle.

Three months into recovery, another surprise hit: my hair started to fall out. It was like each month uncovered a new hurdle, a fresh reminder of how much sepsis had taken from me. Six months after my initial surgery, I needed a second operation to replace the mesh in my abdomen, which had to be removed the first time due to infection. The anxiety from going back to the hospital for additional surgery was enormous. I cried from the moment I walked through the hospital doors until they put the anesthesia mask on my face. That surgery intensified my healing process all over again, setting me back to square one.

As I struggled to cope with these challenges, I started looking for support online. I stumbled upon Sepsis Alliance, an organization founded by Dr. Carl Flatley in 2007 after his daughter Erin died of sepsis at just 23 years old. I connected with sepsis.org, where I found resources, a community, and a glimmer of hope. This organization raises awareness for sepsis, reaching out to the public and healthcare professionals. It was a lifeline when I felt isolated, a reminder that others were going through this, too.

A year into my recovery, I finally decided to seek counseling. I found a compassionate therapist who, although he didn't specialize in PTSD, and while he wasn't local, was exactly what I needed. We worked through my experiences, and he helped me process the trauma that came with each sepsis episode. He also helped me imagine my new life with new roadblocks and opportunities.

When Sepsis Alliance Connect launched a program specifically for survivors, I didn't hesitate—I volunteered right away. They were forming support groups for sepsis survivors, caregivers, and those who'd lost loved ones to sepsis. I trained as a facilitator, and now, every other Thursday, I lead a group on Zoom for fellow survivors. That group has been the single greatest healing experience of my life. I get as much out of it as those who attend, watching us find strength in shared stories and understanding.

Years later, I still live with post-sepsis syndrome, a constant reminder of the battle my body has endured. Sepsis didn't just come and go—it left scars that reveal themselves every day in new ways. I've developed more health issues from the recurring infections, the organ damage, and the heavy doses of antibiotics and vasopressors. It feels like every week brings a new challenge to face, a fresh problem to address. But I keep going, finding ways to help others and draw strength from the support around me.

26   SANDRA KLEIER

KEY TAKEAWAYS

➤ Recognizing the stages of sepsis can be life-saving; acting on initial signs like fever, rapid breathing, and fatigue is critical before the condition worsens.

➤ Severe sepsis brings alarming symptoms, including organ dysfunction and dangerous blood pressure drops; swift medical intervention is essential at this stage.

➤ Septic shock, the final and most severe stage, requires immediate, life-saving measures due to life-threatening blood pressure drops and failing organs.

➤ Know your body's warning signs and respond quickly—trusting these signs and seeking help without delay can make a big difference.

➤ Support networks and education, like those provided by Sepsis Alliance, offer resources for both sepsis survivors and healthcare providers to understand post-sepsis challenges.

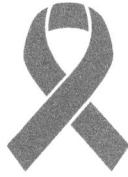

CHAPTER THREE

THE ICU EXPERIENCE FROM A PATIENT'S PERSPECTIVE

One day, you might find yourself or a loved one in the ICU, and I want to make that experience less overwhelming or frightening. The ICU is intimidating with its machines, alarms, and constant activity. But understanding what to expect can help you feel more prepared and less alone.

The first thing I remember after waking up in the ICU was seeing my husband and daughters holding my hands. My husband squeezed my hand and asked me to squeeze back, but I couldn't move. Panic set in, but I didn't want him to see my fear—I wanted him to know I was okay. We had recently watched a movie where a couple communicates by blinking, so I started blinking in response to his questions, hoping he'd catch on. He didn't.

Later, I woke again to find a calm male nurse by my side. He explained where I was and what had happened. Then he told me I was in Room #13. I'm not superstitious, but that number gave me pause! Still, his gentle explanation reassured me. I desperately wanted to ask questions, but I didn't have the strength—or the means—to communicate.

When they woke me fully the next day, I was still on a ventilator, and communicating became a new challenge. At first, I tried spelling out letters in the air, but the nurses struggled to guess what I was saying. Finally, I asked for paper to draw pictures or write notes. Eventually, they found a whiteboard that already had taped letters on it for another purpose, but it had just enough space for me to scribble messages.

The Ice Storm That Changed Everything

I entered the hospital on December 19, 2013, and had surgery the next day. A massive ice storm swept through Kansas by Friday night, stranding my family at home and the hospital staff on-site. Nurses and doctors who didn't live nearby stayed overnight at the hospital, unable to leave. It was during this time that I grew incredibly close to the staff.

After the ice storm, we were hit by a huge snowfall, and I joked that they should go outside and make snow angels. The ICU rooms surrounded an outdoor courtyard, so the staff moved my bed close to the window and raised it high so I could see outside. To my delight, the nurses, respiratory therapists, and even a few doctors went outside and made snow angels just for me. That moment—watching them laugh and play in the snow—was the highlight of my ICU stay.

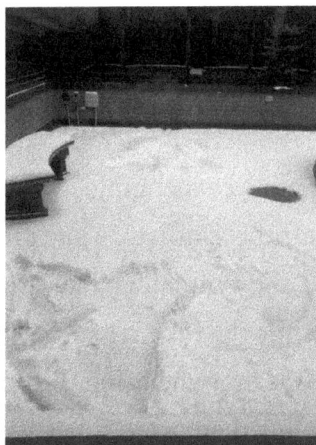

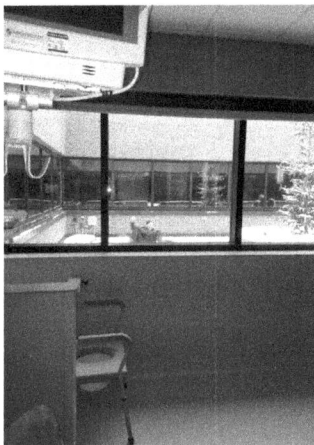

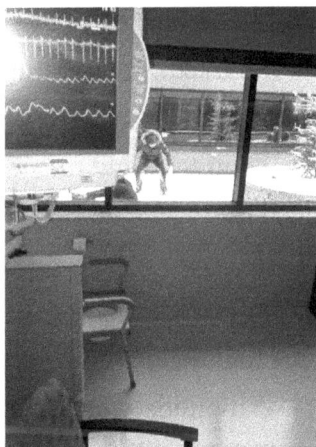

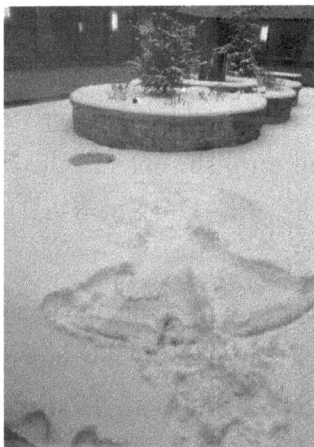

Surprisingly, I found the ICU to be a comforting place. There was always someone at my bedside, ready to explain every beep and alarm. They cared for me as an individual, and

I never felt alone, even when the weather kept my family away. Of course, there were periods of loneliness, but the staff filled the void. Once I was awake, I passed the time on Facebook. Friends teased me, saying I couldn't be that sick if I were online, but I reminded them—I was still on a ventilator!

The Hardest Moments

Three moments stand out as the most challenging.

The first was being weaned off the ventilator. The process was terrifying. The staff lowered the ventilator's rate, forcing me to breathe more on my own while the tube remained in my lungs. The sensation of choking was overwhelming. Breathing slowly through my nose helped, but there were times when I panicked. I hit the call light during a particularly bad moment, and the unit supervisor answered. She asked, "How can I help you?" As I couldn't answer while intubated, I banged on the bedrail until she entered the room, coming to my rescue. She quickly calmed me down and guided me to a regular breathing rhythm.

The second challenge was standing and sitting for the first time. Because of my low blood pressure, the medical staff had resuscitated me with IV fluids—45 pounds worth. At just 5'1", the extra weight made me feel like a cow (no offense to cows). Sitting in a chair was exhausting, and walking behind a wheelchair felt like climbing a mountain. By the time I was discharged from the ICU on December 22, walking even a few steps felt like the hardest thing I'd ever done.

The final hurdle was leaving the ICU's one-on-one care. In the ICU, someone was always there. On the medical floor, I was one of six patients. My vital signs were checked every 4 hours instead of every 15 minutes like they had been, and responses to the call light came when someone had time. The care was still good, but the transition was a brutal wake-up call.

Family in the Eye of the Storm

My husband, Ron, was my rock during those ICU days, though the weight of the situation was heavy on him. Ron looks back at it and says, "Everyone was extremely concerned about the seriousness of her condition. Some family members didn't fully understand the seriousness and recovery period for septic shock. It was helpful that a surgeon and a couple of nurses informed us she had a severe case and it may take 6 months to reach mostly recovered."

Hearing those words didn't make it easier for Ron, but knowing what to expect gave him some direction. He stayed by my side, doing everything he could to let me know he was there, even when I couldn't respond.

My oldest daughter, Jessica, is an RN, and having her medical background was invaluable. "Having other family around helped for comfort and support," she said. "But what made the biggest difference was staying in constant communication with the doctors and nurses, keeping everyone updated."

For Jessica, knowledge was power. Understanding what was

happening medically gave her some control in a situation that felt otherwise uncontrollable. She prayed often, though, as she admits, "Not nearly as much as I do now."

My middle daughter, Melanie, had a different experience. She wasn't the one asking medical questions or deciphering updates; she was the one waiting. And waiting is its own kind of torment. "I don't remember doing anything specific to cope," she said. "I just sat there, waiting for any news and dealing with the anxiety."

Melanie shared that the presence of family was her lifeline during those uncertain days. "The waiting was probably the worst part because there's nothing you can do. Having Jess there to navigate the medical stuff and explain things helped relieve some stress."

My youngest daughter, Brooklyn, said, "I coped by leaning on Jess and Mel for support, along with my close friends. It really helps that I have friends who care and are supportive. I prayed a lot. Hearing what the doctors had to say helped with my anxiety and stress. But I'll tell you, seeing you in the ICU, not knowing what the outcome was going to be, really devastated me. And being there before you went into your spine surgery and hearing you tell the doctor that you're not ready to die was heartbreaking. I, for one, am not ready to lose you."

Through their reflections, I learned that my ICU stay wasn't just my battle—it was theirs, too. They coped in their own ways, relying on each other and leaning on the medical team for clarity and comfort. The waiting, the uncertainty, and the sheer helplessness are often overlooked parts of a family's ICU experience, but they are as real and challenging as the physical battles happening inside those walls.

A Message to Patients, Families, and Healthcare Providers

My advice for healthcare providers who dedicate themselves to the ICU is to prioritize communication. Keep an open line with both patients and their families because you are often their only source of comfort. Honesty matters, but so does clarity—leave the medical jargon outside the room and meet us where we are.

Remember the small details. Even seemingly harmless things, like fragrances, can feel overwhelming for sick patients. My discharge nurse and I discovered that her heavily perfumed fabric softener was the culprit of my nausea and headache. When I gently mentioned the nauseating odor, she was open to the feedback, and it became a lesson for both of us. It's a reminder to approach these conversations with kindness and understanding, as they are often opportunities for growth and connection.

For those in the ICU or supporting a loved one there, never hesitate to speak up. Your voice matters, whether asking a question, voicing a concern, or addressing discomfort. Just as the ICU staff is there to care for you, you have a role in advocating for yourself or your loved one.

And finally, recognize that while the ICU is a place of intense challenges, it's also a place where human connection shines. From snow angels in the courtyard to a kind nurse calming a panicked moment, those little acts of compassion remind us that even in our most vulnerable moments, we are not alone.

KEY TAKEAWAYS

➤ The ICU can be overwhelming, but understanding what to expect can help ease the fear and uncertainty for patients and their families.

➤ Communication, whether through blinking, writing, or finding creative methods like a whiteboard, is vital for expressing needs and maintaining a connection when words fail.

➤ Moments of human connection, like nurses making snow angels or calm reassurances during panic, can transform the ICU experience into one of comfort and hope.

➤ Families face their own battles of waiting, uncertainty, and helplessness, but staying informed, leaning on each other, and maintaining open communication with medical staff can provide strength and clarity.

➤ Advocating for yourself or a loved one in the ICU, addressing discomforts, and valuing small acts of kindness can make a profound difference in navigating this challenging time.

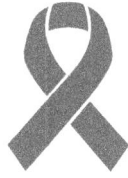

CHAPTER FOUR

RECOVERY MILESTONES: 1, 5, 10 YEARS

Recovering from sepsis is not a straight path. It's full of twists, setbacks, and unexpected detours. And even though doctors might tell you, "You're lucky to be alive," what they don't tell you is how hard it is to *live* after sepsis. The physical exhaustion, the emotional turmoil, and the uncertainty about what the future holds all add up to an overwhelming experience.

This chapter is about those milestones—one year, five years, and ten years out from sepsis. It's about what recovery looks like medically, emotionally, and mentally. I want to share what I went through, what I learned, and what others have told me about their recoveries. You *can* recover, even if it doesn't feel like it right now. Your life may not go back to what it was before, but that doesn't mean it can't still be meaningful and fulfilling.

The First Year

That first year was *brutal*. My emotions swung wildly—I would go from feeling grateful to be alive to being completely overwhelmed with depression. Some days, I genuinely wondered if I would ever heal.

The physical side of recovery was just as tough. I was exhausted *all the time*. It took everything in me just to get out of bed in the morning, and by the time I was up, I already needed a nap. The fatigue, the pain, and the weakness made me feel like I was trapped in a body that wasn't mine anymore. And then, just when I thought I might be making progress, I had to have another surgery six months after my bowel perforation and septic shock. It felt like I couldn't catch a break. My body was fragile, and my spirit was shattered.

At one year out, I realized something had to change. I knew I had PTSD and that I needed help, but in Kansas City, no one specialized in PTSD for sepsis survivors besides the VA (Veterans Association). Still, I found a counselor. He didn't specialize in PTSD, but he did help me understand my anxiety and depression. He helped me see that my life wasn't *over*—it was just *different*. I could redefine who I was. I could use what I had been through to help others.

One thing I've heard from so many other survivors is how

terrifying that first anniversary can be. It's like this looming shadow—what if I get sick again? What if my body fails me *again*? Will I feel this way forever? If you're approaching your one-year mark and feeling that same panic, know it's completely normal. And if you've already passed it, you probably experienced a sense of relief. It doesn't mean all the anxiety disappears, but it does mean you've proven to yourself that you *can* keep going. Many of us find that the fear will lessen.

How to Stay Motivated in Year One:

- Take it one day at a time. Don't look too far ahead—just focus on getting through today.
- Connect with other survivors. Hearing from people who've been where you are can remind you that you're not alone.
- Acknowledge small victories. Maybe you walked a little farther today. Perhaps you got through the day without a panic attack. Every step counts.
- Let yourself feel everything. The fear, relief, and exhaustion are all part of healing.

The Five-Year Mark

For me, the five-year mark was about trying to figure out what I was supposed to do with my life now. Sepsis had left me with so many lingering health issues that returning to a "normal" career wasn't an option. My body needed frequent rest breaks.

My focus was unreliable—I'd start one task, get distracted, and end up halfway through something else without realizing it. It was frustrating for me, and I know it was frustrating for my family, too.

Five years is supposed to feel like a victory—a turning point where you can look back and say, *I made it.* But it didn't feel like progress because, at that point, I had already faced my *fifth* sepsis infection. So instead of reflecting on how far I had come, I was right back in survival mode.

As I write this in February 2025, I feel like I'm still chasing the idea of stability. It's been *three years* since my last infection, yet I still live with that lingering fear. Any time I don't feel well, my mind immediately goes there—*Is this it? Is it happening again?* This past week, I ran a low-grade fever for two days, shivering and dealing with aches, pains, and teeth chattering. That was after a brutal round of norovirus ran through my entire household, and they exhibited the very same symptoms. And yet, I told myself it was just a virus, a rough week.

Fast forward to February 27, 2025—I'm in the hospital again. My *thirteenth* battle with sepsis. Even saying that number out loud feels surreal. Thirteen times. Thirteen fights for my life. This time was different, though. It didn't start the way my previous infections had. The fever wasn't the same—it didn't quickly climb the way it had before. It only lasted two days. That should have been reassuring, right? But there was something else, something I didn't recognize at first.

My level of consciousness was off. I was falling asleep in the middle of tasks, literally standing up and just falling asleep.

I would wake up on the floor, confused. I was unable to take care of myself, unable to push fluids through my tubing, unable even to recognize the danger I was in.

I kept telling myself, *I'm just tired. I just need to rest.* But my husband and my daughter, the RN, knew better. They saw what I couldn't see: that I was declining. I was too weak to make the call for help, so Jessica made it for me. She overrode my stubbornness, picked up the phone, and called an ambulance.

I wasn't happy about it. I fought her on it. But looking back, I know that she saved my life that night. You don't always recognize how sick you are. You can't always trust yourself to see the warning signs, especially after surviving something as traumatic as sepsis. That's why you need people around you who know what to look for. You need people who will step in and say, *You're not okay, and I'm not waiting for you to admit it.* If your gut tells you something is off, listen to it. And if you're too tired, too weak, or too stubborn to listen—let someone else do it for you.

The Ten-Year Mark

I always counted my first septic shock episode December 19, 2013— as my original "anniversary." But then, after each new infection, I felt like I had to reset the clock. My last infection was three years ago, so in my mind, I wasn't really at the ten-year mark anymore—I was at three years post-sepsis *again*. And now, after this most recent infection, I suppose I have to restart the clock *yet again*.

Somewhere around my sixth or seventh anniversary of surviving my 2013 septic shock, something shifted. In the early years, December 19th was a heavy date for me. I dreaded it, relived it, grieved it. But then, one year, something odd happened—I realized the date was coming up, but when the actual day arrived, I forgot all about it.

That was a good feeling. It meant I was no longer grieving that day. I wasn't waking up on December 19th feeling the weight of what happened. It wasn't until afterward that I would remember—*Oh, that was the day. And I survived it.* That realization brought gratitude instead of grief.

When you've had sepsis as many times as I have, milestones don't feel like they used to. There are too many dates. Too many hospital stays. I barely remember the dates of my infections between December 2013 and January 2022. At some point, they just blur together.

If I had only experienced sepsis that one time in 2013, I imagine I'd feel a lot differently today. I'd probably be celebrating being nearly twelve years out, like I conquered something major. And I did—I survived a day that almost took my life. But survival wasn't a one-time thing for me. It became a way of life.

What Really Matters

I don't celebrate anniversaries anymore. I don't count the years the way I used to. But what I *do* celebrate is the fact that I'm still here. No matter what condition I'm in, no matter how many times I've had to fight for my life—I am still here. And that means I get to keep doing the things that bring me joy. I get to spend time with my children and grandchildren. I get to share my story. I get to wake up every day and make the choice to keep moving forward.

If you're reading this and struggling to make sense of your own milestones, know this: It's okay if your journey doesn't look like anyone else's. It's okay if your recovery doesn't follow a neat, linear path. And as long as you're here, you still have a life to live.

Moving Forward, One Day at a Time

Over the years, I've learned that no two recoveries look the same. Some survivors make it to their milestones with few complications, while others—like me—find themselves re-starting the clock over and over again. But wherever you are in your journey, one thing remains true: you are not alone. One of the hardest parts of recovery is the feeling that no one else understands. Sepsis is still so widely misunderstood, even in the medical world, which makes it even harder to explain to friends and family. But I promise you—there *are* people who understand. Having a support system, whether a family member, a friend, or an online survivor community, can make all the difference.

I worry most for those who don't have that support. Older people, in particular, suffer not just physically but emotionally. Many of them are isolated and don't have the technical skills to go online and find resources or connect with other survivors. They're left to navigate this terrifying experience on their own, and that's something that needs to change.

Finding Strength in the Setbacks

I won't pretend every milestone has felt like a victory. At the five-year mark, I was facing my fifth sepsis infection. And now, after three years sepsis-free, I thought I had finally broken the cycle—only to find myself back in the hospital, starting over again. It's frustrating. It's heartbreaking. But it's not the end.

No matter how many times I've had to reset my timeline, I refuse to give up. I believe I will reach five years sepsis-free. I hope I will make it to ten. And if I have to start over again, I will. I *will* keep moving forward.

If you're just starting your recovery, my biggest advice is to take one day at a time. That's it. Just focus on getting through *today*. At the end of each day, write down a little note about how you felt, what you did, or any small progress you made. It doesn't have to be much—just a sentence or two. And on the hard days, when you feel like you're stuck, those little notes will remind you that you *are* moving forward, even when it doesn't feel like it. Over time, you'll be able to look back and see just how far you've come.

KEY TAKEAWAYS

➢ Recovery from sepsis is not linear—setbacks are common, but they don't erase progress. Each milestone, whether one year, five years, or ten, brings its own challenges and lessons.

➢ The first year is often the hardest, filled with extreme fatigue, emotional turmoil, and PTSD, but finding support and focusing on small victories can make a difference.

➢ Milestones don't always feel celebratory—when survival becomes a way of life, the focus shifts from counting years to appreciating the moments that matter.

➢ Even when your journey resets, persistence is everything—taking it one day at a time, leaning on a support system, and refusing to give up is what makes recovery possible.

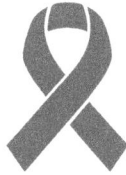

CHAPTER FIVE

POST-SEPSIS SYNDROME: A NEW BEGINNING

No one talks about what happens *after* you survive sepsis. Everyone around you is just so relieved that you're alive. But surviving is just the beginning. I never imagined how much of a toll it would take on me mentally, emotionally, and physically. I thought I'd bounce back the way I always had before. I thought I was strong, tough, and determined enough. But Post-Sepsis Syndrome had other plans.

I'm sharing this with you now because if you're in this phase of recovery, you deserve to know you're not crazy and you're definitely not alone. Post-Sepsis Syndrome is real, and it changes everything. But there's still hope. This is what it looked like for me.

My surgeon warned me that recovery would take longer than my previous surgeries, but nothing could've prepared me for the mind-numbing fatigue that followed. This was not found in any literature I ever came across.

And then came the hair loss.

No one warned me about that, either. As a middle-aged woman, it was devastating. I lost the entire front part of my hairline. It receded almost all the way back to my ears. And the rest of my hair was so thin. I became so self-conscious that I started wearing wigs. Thankfully, synthetic wigs have come a long way, and they're affordable too. I ended up buying several styles so that I could play around and try to feel like myself again.

My New Normal

After my first bout of septic shock, which was caused by a perforated bowel, I was so weak I couldn't even sleep in a regular bed. I needed a hospital bed at home with bed rails just to get out of bed. I couldn't walk without a walker. Mornings were a process. Before I even attempted to get out of bed, I'd take a pain pill. My sweet husband would bring me a cup of coffee while I waited for the medicine to kick in. It usually took about an hour before I felt like I could even get up and go to the bathroom.

Just brushing my teeth and washing my face were major tasks. I had to do it all at the sink, sitting down on my walker.

Washing my hair also happened in the sink, as it used less energy than a full shower. I had to dry my hair sitting down, and I could only manage a full shower once a week, depending on how much energy I had. I even kept my makeup in my bedside table so I could put it on while lying down. I just wanted to feel somewhat human again.

My afternoons were spent napping, reading, or attending doctor appointments. Then it was supper, and I went back to bed to watch TV until I fell asleep. That was my life—day in, day out.

Before sepsis, I was confident and independent. I didn't need anyone or anything. I was used to handling life on my terms. Then, suddenly, I couldn't get out of bed without help. I needed assistance with everything: walking, eating, washing my hair, doing laundry, making meals. I couldn't even do the one thing that I loved most: read. I'd pick up a book, and next thing I knew, I'd fallen asleep. So I stopped trying and just turned on the TV. Driving was out of the question.

My family was supportive. They were kind and sympathetic; they tried their best to help. But the truth is, they couldn't possibly understand what I was going through—not fully. They saw the physical struggles, but I kept the emotional part buried. I didn't want them to see how broken I felt inside. How embarrassed I was of the person I had become. Because when your body doesn't work the way it used to, you start to question who you are. You grieve the version of yourself that used to be, and that grief doesn't come with a timeline.

Feeling Invisible

In 2013, I was hospitalized and fighting for my life. I remember feeling scared, confused, and completely vulnerable. One of the most baffling parts of that experience was realizing my general practitioner, someone I'd known and trusted for years, never came to see me. This was a woman I respected, someone I had worked with professionally, someone I thought would show up in my moment of crisis. But she didn't.

No one told me that the hospital was transitioning to a hospitalist model. No one explained that general practitioners no longer made hospital rounds. So I lay there, waiting and wondering, trying to understand why the doctor who had always been there for me suddenly wasn't.

Eventually, I figured it out on my own. That feeling of being left behind by the very people you're supposed to trust still disturbs me.

The first real support I received was from my general surgeon. We had a long-standing doctor-patient relationship, and he did try to prepare me. He told me it would take at least six months to recover. That alone helped me temper my expectations a little. But looking back, he never once used the words "sepsis" or "septic shock."

And while his intentions were good, I'm convinced that most medical professionals still don't fully understand what recovery from sepsis really looks like. It's not a matter of weeks. It's not just a physical healing process. It changes everything—your body, your mind, your confidence, your identity.

My general practitioner was empathetic. I know she cared. But once again, there was this gap—this lack of understanding. It was as if I were speaking a language that no one around me could understand.

Over the past decade, I've come to know and respect my infectious disease specialist. We've built a rapport. But even then, I've received no roadmap for what to expect during recovery. So, I've made it my mission to educate them.

Yes, *them*. Every doctor, nurse, tech, or specialist I encounter. I bring them articles written specifically for healthcare providers. I try to explain the challenges we face as sepsis survivors, not just the fatigue and brain fog but the emotional fallout, too. And what do I get in return?

Blank stares. Shrugs. The materials I hand over are often set aside and never looked at again. It's like they're more comfortable treating the invading bacteria than acknowledging the patient who's still reeling from the trauma it caused.

We deserve more than to be forgotten the moment we're discharged. My ultimate goal, and maybe yours, too, is to break through that wall of indifference. To speak up, to educate, and to finally be heard.

Showing up for Myself

No one is going to do the work for you. Recovery isn't something your doctors manage. It's something *you* have to face every day. I had to figure that out the hard way. The one thing that saved me was persistence. I had to keep showing up for myself, even on the days I didn't want to. I had to remind myself constantly: one bad day doesn't mean every day will be bad.

I've never been the "poor me" type. I don't ask, "Why me?" I ask, "Why *not* me?" Who am I to think I should be exempt from hardship? There's always someone out there who's worse off, physically or mentally. That perspective kept me grounded.

One of the most surprising gifts that came out of surviving sepsis is the reminder that I'm still *me*. Yes, my physical body was broken. Yes, I was fragile in ways I'd never known before. But deep down, I was still the determined woman I've always been.

Before I developed sepsis, I was a leader at work, in life, and in my community. But after that cold December day, when everything changed, I lost that mojo. It was as if a part of me had gone dormant. But slowly, through participating in focus groups and later facilitating support groups, I started to feel like myself again. Those moments of connection gave me what I needed. They reminded me that I had something valuable to offer and that my voice and experience could help others. And in helping them, I began to heal.

Small Steps, Big Difference

Post-Sepsis Syndrome took a lot from me. But it also gave me the chance to rebuild my purpose and my resilience. There wasn't a single fix or magic solution that helped me get my life back after sepsis. It was the daily little choices that made a difference. And I want to share some of them with you, not because they'll work the same way for everyone, but because they just might offer a place to start.

- I began eating a healthier diet: high in protein and healthy saturated fats, low in carbs, with plenty of fruits, vegetables, and water to help decrease inflammation and boost my immune system. *(Of course, talk to your doctor, especially if you have kidney disease or diabetes, before making major changes.)*

- I rested a lot. And I let myself rest without guilt. Your body and your soul both need time to heal.

- I moved just a little at first. A few leg lifts. A few extra steps. I built up slowly and gave myself grace on the hard days.

- I stuck to a routine as best I could. It gave me structure and a sense of control when everything else felt chaotic.

- I found support. Whether it was online through Sepsis Alliance Connect or just a phone call with someone who truly *got it*, I made sure not to isolate myself.

- I educated myself. Sepsis Alliance offers valuable resources for survivors and provides helpful information to explain this experience to your healthcare providers.

- And yes, I had fun with wigs. Losing your hair is a tough blow, but it doesn't have to steal your joy.

You May Never Be the Same—and That's Okay

If you're reading this and wondering if you'll ever feel "normal" again, let me say this with all the love and truth I can offer: Your new normal is likely going to change. What feels like normal today might not be normal in a month or a year. You may never go back to the version of "normal" you had before sepsis. But that doesn't mean you're lost. It means you're becoming someone new.

For me, although I still maintain my nursing license, my nursing career is over. After 34 years of caring for others, that identity was a huge part of who I was. Letting it go was heartbreaking. But I also realized it wasn't the only way I could make a difference. I joined Sepsis Alliance. I started speaking up, educating both professionals and survivors. I ran for treasurer of our local township. I now serve as treasurer on a scholarship committee for my high school alma mater. I'm even going to run for the school board this Fall (*Eek!*)

All of this, combined with caring for my mother, who lives with us and is battling vascular dementia, has given me purpose. It keeps me from spiraling into sadness or self-pity, even on days when trudging on is the last thing I feel like doing.

Post-Sepsis Syndrome can feel like a cruel joke after everything you've already survived. But if I've learned anything, it's that we get to define what healing looks like. We get to decide what strength looks like. And even if your body isn't what it once was, your spirit—*your will*—can be stronger than ever.

Keep going. Rest when you need to. Laugh when you can. Find a purpose where you least expect it. And never stop fighting for the life you *still* get to live. You're here for a reason. And you are needed.

KEY TAKEAWAYS

➤ Surviving sepsis is just the beginning; Post-Sepsis Syndrome is real, life-altering, and often invisible to those around you.

➤ Recovery is not a linear process and is rarely understood by medical professionals, making it vital to advocate for yourself and educate others.

➤ You may grieve the loss of who you once were, but reclaiming your identity, piece by piece is possible through support, routine, and small daily actions.

➤ Healing is a mix of grace, persistence, and choosing joy in unexpected ways, even if it's through a good wig and a moment of laughter.

➤ Your "new normal" may look different than before, but you still have value, purpose, and a voice that matters.

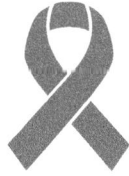

CHAPTER SIX

STORIES OF RESILIENCE: VOICES OF SEPSIS SURVIVORS

I'm Don Smith, and I live in Colorado Springs, CO, USA, and I'm a sepsis survivor.

On Monday, December 18, 2017, my wife, Karen, was having stomach discomfort. During the day, as she got worse, it became likely that she had appendicitis, so I took her to a nearby hospital. Staff there confirmed the diagnosis and scheduled her for surgery that evening. While she waited in the Emergency Department, I ran out to the car to get something and noticed that my right foot hurt. I didn't remember doing anything to it, but I was running a lot then (about 20 miles/

week), so I figured I had strained something. My focus was on Karen, so I didn't think much more about it. Her surgery was successful, and I went home to bed.

On Tuesday, my foot hurt more, and I was feeling tired. I tried using crutches, but I was very clumsy on them. I've been on crutches several times in my life and was surprised to have any problems. Karen came home that night. When I woke up on Wednesday, the pain in my foot was worse, so I decided to go to the doctor. Since my foot hurt, I went to a podiatrist, who misdiagnosed me with gout and gave me some prescriptions to make me more comfortable. At least the painkiller helped some.

When I woke up on Thursday, the pain was worse and I was very weak - so weak that I couldn't get out of bed by myself. As the day went on, I kept feeling worse, and that afternoon Karen and our daughter Marya decided that I needed to go to the hospital - the same one Karen had been in earlier that week. They ran multiple tests and decided to admit me. In my hospital records, there's a diagnosis of sepsis that day, but they didn't tell Karen that. If they told me, I don't remember. I don't remember anything about that day except that I felt worse than I had ever felt in my life, and I didn't know what was wrong or what to do about it.

Early Friday morning, the hospital staff moved me to Intensive Care because I was so sick. That morning, the chief trauma surgeon came in to see me. He told me that I had a severe case of sepsis, that they would take me for surgery as soon as they could get an operating room ready, and that I might not survive the surgery or I might lose my right leg, depending on what they found. Within 30 minutes, I was in an OR for a 2-hour procedure while Karen and Marya waited anxiously. In that surgery, the doctors took tissue samples to send to the lab to determine what kind of infection I had. They also removed skin and other tissue from my right foot and leg. The lab determined that the infection was Strep A, and that I did not have necrotizing fasciitis, so amputation was not required. I survived the surgery and kept my leg, but the doctors put me in a medically-induced coma and on a ventilator. My liver and kidneys failed, and my blood pressure dropped to 60/46. Blood flow to my extremities was weak. I coded at least once. I was very fortunate to survive. I stayed in a coma for 13 days. I missed Christmas and New Year's Day.

I started showing some improvement after Christmas, and on January 3, I came out of the coma to stay after a couple of false starts. When I woke up, I was so weak that I couldn't move except to move my head side to side slightly. Later that day, I started moving my hands, but I couldn't control them very well. I couldn't talk because of the tracheostomy tube in my neck that connected to the ventilator so that I could breathe adequately. So I was awake, but I couldn't move and couldn't talk. Karen told me that I had had sepsis, but I didn't know what that meant. I had heard the word before but had no understanding beyond that. She also showed me my feet, where many of my toes were black and shrunken, and my leg, where I had lost tissue and had wound vacuums attached to help with healing. She told me that it was likely that I would lose some of my toes. I understood (sort of - as much as my addled brain could grasp) but didn't really know how to process that information.

On January 5, surgeons removed the three middle toes from my right foot, along with additional tissue from the top of my foot, including some tendons.

On January 8, I had the trach tube replaced with a smaller tube that had a speaking valve, so I could start talking again. That was a great relief for all of us. That day, I also passed a swallow test and was allowed to start eating. Eating came very slowly. At first, I could only eat 3 or 4 bites at a time because my stomach had shrunk so much. I continued my recovery and began to regain a little bit of strength.

On January 13, the insurance company decided that I could no longer stay in the ICU and that I needed to move to a regular floor at the hospital. That felt like progress to me, but we had to adjust to the lower level of care.

January 17 was the worst day of the entire hospitalization for me, since I have no memory of the first day in the hospital. Surgery was scheduled for 3:00 to remove toes from my left foot. The doctors weren't sure if they would be able to save any of the toes and felt that they might need to remove part of the foot as well. I couldn't eat after 7:00 in the morning to prepare for surgery. The operation was delayed multiple times, and my anxiety became worse and worse and worse. Finally, I had surgery at 7:30 PM after not eating all day. The surgery was successful - 4 dead toes were removed, but the big toe was saved as well as all of my foot. After I was back in my room, the anesthetic began to wear off, and the pain was very intense. After more painkillers were given, I was able to relax and go to sleep.

On January 20, the insurance company decided that I needed to leave. Fortunately, they approved me to go to the rehabilitation floor at the downtown hospital that is connected to the one where I had been for a month. I got very good therapy support, both physical and occupational, and my recovery continued. I had my final major surgery on January 26. This was skin graft surgery to cover the open areas on my right leg and foot. That surgery was a complete success, and the grafts began to heal.

On February 1, I stood for the first time, holding on to parallel bars and balancing on my left heel since my right foot wasn't weight-bearing yet.

Finally, on February 12, I came home from the hospital after almost 2 months. I still wasn't walking, and wouldn't for two more weeks. But I was home and ecstatic to be there.

I still struggle with several things. I have less energy and stamina than I did before sepsis. I get tired more easily from less exertion, and it takes me longer to recover my energy if I have become too tired. I have to plan my activities carefully to avoid getting too tired. I get cold more easily, and once I am cold, it takes longer to warm back up. My memory is much worse. Both short-term and long-term memory are reduced. My ability to analyze and think through things is significantly reduced. I struggle to keep my weight down. I eat half to two-thirds of what I ate before sepsis, and I still struggle. And, of course, I struggle with the limitations imposed by losing most of my toes and having neuropathy in both feet.

My advice for a new survivor is to acknowledge that one

can't go through an experience like this and not be changed. Expect to find changes, physically, mentally, and emotionally. Embrace them and learn who you are now as you continue to work hard to make the best of it.

Sunshine Turns to Septic Shock

I'm Myrna Pair, a sepsis survivor and sepsis advocate, from Everett, WA.

It was May 13, 2020. COVID-19 lockdown and a requirement to mask up everywhere. Outside, it was a glorious sunny spring day, warm enough not to need a jacket. I really didn't feel like walking to Starbucks, but I did so to share time with my daughter. Later, walking to and from Starbucks, we picked up our pre-ordered cold drinks while talking, laughing, enjoying our cool beverages, and soaking up the sunshine on our way home. Such a special time. It is a memory I will always cherish - completely unaware my life would forever change.

A couple of hours after our walk, I experienced diarrhea, but unlike anything I'd experienced before. It was dark, like used coffee grounds, with a putrid smell. Later, I vomited, and it resembled the diarrhea I'd had as well as its smell. I thought the coffee drink disagreed with me, or it was a virus. I had no idea this kind of diarrhea signaled gastrointestinal bleeding! I learned about that weeks later.

After 13 hours, I was weak and dehydrated. My daughter called 911. The EMTs transported me to the Emergency

Department (ED). Within minutes of arriving at the ED, blood tests, fluid resuscitation, and an ECG began. Then a portable chest X-ray showed borderline vascular congestion, and a portable abdominal CT found pancolitis. More blood tests were ordered and completed. Three sepsis early warning score systems (qSOFA, MEWS, and NEWS) tracked my vital signs. Emergent exploratory abdominal surgery took place approximately four hours later, resulting in the removal of my colon. An ileostomy was constructed, routing the end of my small intestine (the stoma) through an opening in my abdomen, diverting waste into a pouch secured with an adhesive wafer. No one knows why my colon became infected; it just did.

Eight days later, I was discharged and found I'd lost 28 pounds. Initially, the primary sepsis symptom was experienced as a teeth-chattering cold. In hindsight, confusion (I was not thinking logically) and shortness of breath (very hard to holler for help) would be considered symptoms. I didn't know what the symptoms of sepsis included. I didn't know what sepsis was! I only knew that it wasn't something good. I thought my symptoms were from dehydration, nothing more.

Since 2020, two surgeries have occurred. An ostomy reversal in 2021, and in 2024, open mesh hernia surgery for three incisional hernias and one inguinal hernia. Digestive and bowel issues continue, though they have improved over time. Between 13 and 19 medications and supplements are taken daily. Medical trauma, PTSD, and Post-Sepsis Syndrome remain ongoing challenges. I consider myself extremely fortunate to be alive and pursuing my passion. Driven by my passion to raise sepsis awareness, share its effects, and promote prevention, **BE Sepsis Smart** came to fruition, providing (from a sepsis survivor's perspective) a deeper understanding of sepsis and recovery. Learn more about my story, personal challenges, life today, and the prevention of sepsis.

My Advice to New Sepsis Survivors

- Ask questions. If told you have or had sepsis, ask what sepsis is and what type of sepsis you had (sepsis, severe sepsis, or septic shock). Ask for information and/or resources about sepsis.
- If in the ICU, find out why and what happened that led to the ICU being needed.
- If organs failed, find out if they recovered completely.
- Ask all the questions you can while hospitalized. Or have your advocate ask the questions in the event you are not able.
- If at all possible, have an advocate with you upon arrival at the hospital.
- Order all records - medical, Fire Department EMT, other physicians, or organizations involved in your care.
- Join an advice group (Sepsis Alliance affinity groups, Facebook groups dedicated to sepsis, or other groups specific to any ongoing outcomes or issues).
- Provide your primary care physician (PCP) with information about sepsis (Sepsis Alliance physician letter can be found online).

- Get any referrals from your surgeon or PCP early on when needed. These may include physical therapy, speech therapy, and other tests (MRI, CT, and so on).
- Explain to friends and family any issues resulting from sepsis - brain fog, physical ongoing issues, fatigue, memory issues, your limitations, things you can no longer do, and such. Refer them to the Sepsis Alliance website.
- When able to work or attend school, with some limitations, look into Section 504 accommodations.

Websites:
ostomy.org
sepsis.org
besepsissmart.com

G.M. - Bozeman, Montana

I'm a sepsis survivor.

On December 17, 2023, I had some lower back pain, which I attributed to "overdoing it" as I prepared for a holiday party. The pain increased as the evening progressed. By the next morning, I was so uncomfortable that my husband took me to our local hospital's Emergency Department. They performed a CT scan and an X-ray. The doctor diagnosed a strained lumbar muscle, sent me home with prescriptions for an opioid and a muscle relaxer, and said that I should feel better in a few days.

Over the next five days, I was taken by ambulance twice

and spent 4 days in the hospital. Most of the time, I was in agony, even while taking powerful pain medication. By the evening of the 23rd, I had not been able to urinate since early in the day, my heart rate was fluctuating, sometimes as high as 188, my veins had collapsed, and I'd begun to have convulsions. I was flown by air ambulance to a large regional hospital.

When I arrived, I heard the EMT tell the medical team that my blood pressure was 40/20 and my pulse was 20. A neurosurgeon did emergency spinal surgery to remove two large abscesses from the lumbar region of my spine.

I spent a few days in the ICU and then was transferred to the cardiac floor, where I was on complete bed rest for days. While there, I developed three deep vein blood clots in my legs, probably from lack of movement. I had chest pain one morning; a blood test showed a very high amount of troponin in my system (a protein that can indicate a heart attack). I had a heart catheterization to determine whether there was damage. I didn't have any, and they determined that the high level was probably due to my high, irregular heart rate. The following day, they performed a cardioversion to try to regulate my heart rate. That worked, but for only 23 hours.

I had two more surgeries by the end of January and spent 8 weeks in hospitals. There, I had daily physical therapy and occupational therapy sessions to increase my strength, balance, and stamina. My heart, brain, lungs, pancreas, and liver were all affected to one degree or another. I spent 6 weeks on IV antibiotics and then two more weeks taking them orally. After leaving the hospital, home health nurses came to my house to change my wound-vac and check my progress 3 times a week for 6 weeks.

A year and a half later, I am doing most of the things I could do before sepsis, albeit a little slower and more carefully. My thought process is diminished, but it has come a long way since I left the hospital. The congestive heart failure has reversed itself, my liver enzymes are back in the normal range, and I was able to discontinue oxygen use at the end of April 2024.

My advice to anyone recovering from sepsis is to be patient with yourself and with the healing process. Ask for and accept help when offered. That is something that I was never comfortable with, but it becomes a necessity when it takes 30 minutes to get dressed, and putting socks on unaided is impossible. People brought us meals, which was humbling, but so welcome. Take it a day at a time.

Darrell Raikes, Lebanon, KY

I'm a sepsis survivor.

In the spring of 2015, doctors determined that I needed a partial knee replacement after several unsuccessful knee scopes. On the morning of May 26, I arrived at the hospital, unaware that stepping into the elevator would be my last clear memory for some time.

My wife later recounted that after the surgery, I was able to walk the hallway, enjoy a hamburger, and even text my brother. However, the doctor informed us that my only chance of survival was to be placed on a ventilator. I was told I signed the necessary forms with my wife, but I had no memory of doing so. I was then put on a ventilator and urgently transferred from Good Sam Hospital to the University of Kentucky Hospital. The medical team believed I had experienced an allergic reaction to the anesthesia, which caused my lungs to bleed and ultimately led to septic shock.

As my condition deteriorated, my organs began to fail, including my kidneys and lungs. My right lung collapsed, necessitating a chest tube, and I developed Acute Respiratory Distress Syndrome (ARDS). To prevent blood clots from reaching my heart and lungs, the doctors inserted an inferior vena cava (IVC) filter. Eventually, they determined that a tracheostomy was necessary, marking a critical turning point in my recovery.

When I began to regain consciousness about 20 days later, I realized I had lost all muscle mass and was unable to move or speak. I remained in the ICU until June 30, 2015, holding onto a mix of unforgettable memories—both good and bad. After becoming stable enough, I was transferred to two rehabilitation hospitals for tracheostomy removal and to regain overall strength.

Years later, I still face lingering challenges from this traumatic experience, including PTSD, anxiety, muscle weakness, neuropathy, and other mental health issues. I also have a scarred lung from ARDS, which has affected my breathing.

Throughout this journey, I could not have made it without my family—especially my wife—and the dedicated doctors and staff at the University of Kentucky, particularly Dr. Ashley Montgomery.

Surviving is more than just being alive. It's not about returning to "normal" or meeting the expectations of others. For me, survival means moving forward—creating new memories and leaving the dread behind. The journey can be challenging, with frequent setbacks, but ultimately, it requires putting one foot in front of the other. Determination is key. To truly survive, you must embrace your future and leave the past behind.

Since surviving sepsis, I have traveled across the country to receive several awards, including the International ICU Hero of the Year from the Society of Critical Care Medicine and the Erin K. Flatley Spirit Award from Sepsis Alliance. I have had the privilege of speaking at events such as the American Delirium Society in Boston, the CHEST Convention in New Orleans, and various venues throughout Kentucky. I served on a patient advisory council at UK Hospital and, prior to COVID, volunteered as a mentor for critically ill patients in the ICU. I'm a dedicated advocate for sepsis awareness and a champion for sepsis protocols in Kentucky.

To a new survivor, I would say, "Have patience." It takes the body a long time to heal, but you will eventually get better. You might not ever be the person you were before, but you will get better. Join online groups and search for answers from others who have had a similar experience. Then accept the person you have become, and it's ok to be different. Once you have accepted, go out into the world and make a difference for others.

For more information or to contact me, visit my website: www.ez-caregiver.com.

Anika Pinter, Berlin, Germany

I'm Anika Pinter, and I'm a sepsis survivor.

My sepsis story consists of two parts. The first part is the medical storyline, but this is not what I remember. The second is what I "remember," a crazy mixture of weird spaces, dreams, and hallucinations where my crazy brain took me while sepsis, while in medical coma, and while delirium, and after that. I will give you a little insight into both parts.

*The crazy-brain parts I remember are marked like this to be clear that this is not reality. My sepsis story starts in December 2022. During this time, I was not in my hometown. I was in another city working for three weeks. I stayed in my sister's house for these weeks, and I think this was life-saving for me. It started with a cold. It didn't feel too bad, so I continued working. Suddenly, from one second to the next, it got worse. I tried to continue working, but it got worse. I stopped working, but it still got worse. We went to see a doctor. I could hardly walk to the car, and I needed a wheelchair to make my way from the parking lot to the doctor's.

Surprisingly, the doctor decided that I was fine and told me that my condition was too good for antibiotics. Twelve hours later, my sister called the ambulance because my condition scared her. From then on, my brain disappears from reality. What happens around me: the ambulance doesn't want to take me to the hospital first, but then they do because my condition is getting worse. I can't remember much from the ER. I must stay in the hospital. I have sepsis, pneumonia, my ECG is not okay, and I have neurological issues. I am brought to a hospital floor, which I completely do not remember. I must be somewhere else because I told my sister that I had to reach a ferry while they tested me for brain hemorrhage and tried to help me breathe. I am getting worse. They brought me to the ICU. I will be in a medical coma on a ventilator for the following 8 days.

*I sit in a room in a bed. The room is wrapped in red and green light. The walls are hung with postcards and old items, giving it the look of an old bar. It smells strange. There is another person in the room who is not speaking. Something is not okay here. I have a cable tie on my forehead. To put it more precisely, the cable tie goes through the bone over my eye socket and is fixed to the bed. I think this is interesting because it doesn't hurt. I nod off. My influenza test was positive. To determine the presence of bacteria in the lungs, they must wait for the results of prepared cultures. Because I have none of the typical risk factors for being so ill from pneumonia or influenza, the doctors were convinced that a rare, nasty killer bacterium is inside me. So, they asked my sister all the time if I had been traveling, what I ate, where I was, and more to find out what was trying to kill me. There must be a lot of trouble around me.

*I am in this room again. Red. Green. I can hear people somewhere in the building. Does someone outside know that we are here? I ask myself how you can put a cable tie out of a bone without any tools. I only have brutal ideas. The silent person next to me is not helpful at all. In the real world, my heart is also not in good shape, and my body doesn't like the sepsis therapy, and they still have a lot of questions. Because I seem to be restless in a coma, they give me ketamine.

*Another room. Everything is white. A huge hospital bed. My arms are fixed. The blanket is so heavy that I can't move. It is so quiet that I'm getting scared. I can't move and I can barely breathe. In the real world, they found the bacterium, and it is not the rare killer bacterium they expected. It's just pneumococcus, but with the influenza virus on top, my no-risk-factors body is lying there in the ICU on a ventilator with sepsis.

*The white room. Eternities pass. Did someone forget me here? I can see a cross on a tile hanging on the wall. Upcoming thoughts about dying and death, I try to push aside. Could anybody remove the blanket, please? They change the antibiotics and I'm getting better. They play music and show me voice messages from friends, while my sister hangs paper stars on the walls that my niece made for me for Christmas. My brain is somewhere else. On December 26th, they started to wake me up.

*Delirium. I find myself in a kind of reality show that seems to be shot in a hospital. Cameras are everywhere, filming everything, regardless of any private sphere. There are actors everywhere who claim to be doctors or nurses. I let them know regularly that I see through that. It is incredibly noisy here; I can hear people and machines rushing everywhere. On top of it, it seems to be a very aggressive film set, where people are fired constantly when they make mistakes.

All the time, I am asking myself how I came into this hell. I can't remember the moment I came into that building. When I try to say something, I hear a voice I don't know. I sound like someone who has been screaming for the last 24 hours and has had a lot of alcohol. I am not feeling good. And what the hell is running from all these tubes into my body? I am stressed and not cooperative in the next few days. I remove tubes and needles from my body all the time.

*I start making escape plans out of the hospital show. But I'm sure that this won't be easy. First, I can't stand up for some reason. Second, I have no idea what is outside my room. What kind of building, on which street, in which city? I am staring out of the window to identify something. In real life, I'm still hard to handle. The doctors tell my family that this is normal after a coma and will disappear. In a sepsis group on Facebook, survivors wrote what they remember from coma or delirium. Not a single person was in a nice place in a coma or delirium. Everybody who remembered anything was in hell.

*Another problem is that I'm sure that somebody made digital avatars of my sister and my best friend. So, I always have to check people around me to know if they are real or not. I start asking trick questions with my alcoholic voice to everybody to find that out. I explain to my avatar sister that I know she is not real. My poor sister. After fearing for my life, she now has to listen to all this bullshit that my delirium-brain produces. When delirium is leaving and re-ality is coming, this transition is not instantaneous. I start switching between both worlds. Later, I mix reality with my dreams. All the time, I must ask people if we really had a conversation like this or not. My words are still weird. The reality show and cameras are gone, but my brain continues to have a lot of magic tricks for me. Everybody around me is orange. The skin on my own legs is orange and crumpled. Orange people come in, do something to one of the machines, or prick into my orange skin. An orange physiotherapist wants to practice standing up with me: orange everywhere, orange sister, orange friends. I ask them if they also see all this orange. No. The delirium reality show immediately tries to press a new conspiracy theory about orange people into my thoughts. I try to send it away. I can drink from a feeding cup now, but I cannot put it back on the desk directly in front of me when I don't touch the desk to know where it ends. It seems my brain has lost its spatial awareness for things I see. I hope that it is not like this. I see myself back in the real world running over people who are standing directly in front of me. It would be very unpleasant.

My brain is doing less magic, and I practice walking with the physiotherapist, who is a little less orange every day. There are less tubes and needles in my body. On New Year's Eve, I am lying here listening to the fireworks in the city and thinking that this is really the craziest New Year's Eve I've ever had. The next day, I can move to the normal floor.

At the normal floor, people say things like: "Oh, how good to see you sitting!" and "Do you remember me?" I don't. The bathroom is 15 steps away from my bed. I have never walked this distance alone since I have been here, so I decided that it is a good moment to try this out.

My roommate Marianne is at least 20 years older than I and had a severe heart attack. Compared with me, she looks like a fitness goddess. She googles sepsis and explains to me what I have. This is nice of her, because to be honest, I still don't know much about it at this point.

The day they discharged me from the hospital, I was surprised. I still feel very weak. To change this, I got a place in a rehab hospital. Until it starts, I'll stay with my parents. I couldn't sit for so many hours, and going back home to Berlin isn't an option. My rehab hospital is in a cute village in the black forest. At the reception, there is a sign that says: *Please don't touch the squirrels and foxes.* Okay, I won't.

The rehab hospital was the best thing that could have happened to me, helping me grow from a wobbly jelly into a person who can participate in normal life. Unfortunately, I had to pause being there because I tested positive for COVID, but I could return later and continue rehab. I am grateful for what the therapists there have done for me.

At home. It is February. It would be a lie to say that everything is normal now. I have a collection of weird things and symptoms, and later I learn from lovely people at Sepsis Alliance that this is Post-Sepsis Syndrome. To give you a small insight into my post-sepsis life: my lung function is still bad, I have asthma now, and my heart has something called left bundle branch block, which sounds in German more like football than a diagnosis. My brain is getting much better, but it still has interesting magic surprises for me. I smell things that are not real. The smell from the ICU is in the streets and even in my shampoo. Sometimes, the smell of the green and red coma room visits me for a few seconds, and I find myself touching my forehead where the cable tie was. I cannot use heavy blankets. I lose hair, I am anemic, and my nails and parts of my skin peel in layers. I get dizzy easily, and in winter, I have every stupid virus that goes around and scares me because I know what condition they can bring you. I am not always able to cope with too much stress and pressure anymore, and I get restless quite often.

Some symptoms persist, while others disappear or come and go in waves. Sepsis confuses your entire system; some things can heal, others cannot.

But to be clear, everybody who survives sepsis is one of the lucky ones.

And so I am.

My advice to new sepsis survivors:

- Give your body time; it has accomplished a lot.
- Perhaps you will have a few strange symptoms after sepsis. This is absolutely normal.
- It will take time for you to regain a sense of body confidence, but you can work on it.
- Training can help a lot to recover and feel better– no matter what "training" is for you at the moment.
- Be kind to your body and be kind to yourself - nothing must stay like it is.

Back From the Brink:
My Story of Surviving Septic Shock

Norma Sandor, Sepsis Survivor, Ontario, Canada

ER Visit and Discharge

I suffered septic shock nearly five years ago at 56. When I began showing signs of a urinary tract infection and a kidney stone in early August 2020, I wasn't overly concerned—I'd been through this before. When my urologist couldn't see me for a week, I asked to be placed on a cancellation list.

As my pain escalated to a 9 out of 10, I called an ambulance at 1:00 a.m. on August 5. At the ER, tests confirmed a UTI and a 4mm obstructive kidney stone. Initially, I was told I'd be admitted—what a relief—until plans changed. Without explanation, I was discharged with three prescriptions. The nurses looked uneasy, but I convinced myself the doctor knew best.

At home, I ate just enough to take my meds, drank some water, and lay down, chilled to the bone. I told my husband not to wake me. That night, I drifted in and out of sleep, my muffled cries for help stuck in my throat. I thought I was dreaming—but I was slipping away.

By some miracle, my 75-year-old husband checked on me at 4:30 a.m. and found me unresponsive on the floor. He called close friends for help and phoned an ambulance. I later learned the paramedics struggled to find a viable IV site—I was severely dehydrated. My lips and nail beds were cyanotic, my hands and feet ice cold, and my speech slurred. All signs of sepsis, though I didn't know it yet.

Second ER Visit: Back and Unresponsive

I don't remember returning to the ER, but my records tell the story. I was in septic shock with multi-organ failure—heart, lungs, kidneys, and liver. My blood pressure had plummeted to 46/26, oxygen levels were dangerously low, and my body temperature had dropped to 34.5°C (94.1°F). I was jaundiced, hypoglycemic, and hypotensive despite fluid resuscitation. I was intubated, ventilated, and given vasopressors to preserve blood flow to my brain and organs.

My husband was called to the hospital—not to authorize an ICU transfer, but to say goodbye. Doctors didn't expect me to survive the night.

Transfer, Coma, and ICU

I was rushed to an urban hospital ICU under a "Danger to Life and Limb" protocol. A stent was placed between my kidney and bladder, and a Foley catheter was inserted. I was kept in a medically induced coma as physicians scrambled to save me.

They gave me a 0% chance of survival. My husband was told—over the phone—to prepare for the worst. But I wasn't ready to go. And many were praying.

While awaiting blood culture results, I teetered between life and death. An aggressive antibiotic cocktail was started to fight E. coli and Aerococcus urinae. Though stabilized, I began retaining massive fluid—gaining nearly 70 pounds in days. Jaundiced and unrecognizable, I was isolated for ten days—no visitors—likely due to COVID-19 and my fragile state.

Then, complications multiplied. Fearing kidney failure, I was transferred for dialysis prep. During catheter placement, my carotid artery was accidentally pierced—twice—nearly grazing the aorta. I was rushed to another city hospital, two hours away, where a team of cardiovascular surgeons performed emergency aortic arch repair. (In December 2022, I learned that my vagus nerve had been nicked during surgery, causing paralysis of my left vocal cord.)

While still in a coma, I developed pneumonia from an infected arterial line, a necrotic fingertip, a contractured left hand, hypertrophic scarring, and mottled skin. Once stable, I was transferred back for three weeks of renal therapy. I emerged from the coma in late August.

Waking Up: What Happened?

Waking up was surreal. I didn't know what had happened. My mind was foggy. My body, foreign. I couldn't speak or move. The world felt distorted, like I was underwater, watching from a distance.

I had no memory of the ICU. I awoke in a ward bed, still on oxygen, tube feedings, IV antibiotics, and pain meds. I couldn't eat, talk, or move independently.

Thankfully, I avoided full ICU delirium, though I later recognized a few harmless hallucinations. The nurses were kind and committed, despite working short-staffed during the pandemic.Wound care became a daily struggle. I stubbornly refused pressure sore checks, convinced I had none. Nurses tried with gentle persistence. I made sure they couldn't sneak a peek during bedpan transfers. They joked about who might win me over—but no one ever did.

A childhood friend who worked on the ward cared for me. We reminisced and laughed—her presence, a true gift. My cousins' daughters, who also worked there, visited whenever they could. Their brief drop-ins brought warmth into my sterile world.

One emotional highlight was when my sister wheeled me outside to the hospital courtyard. The sunlight on my face and the soft breeze in my hair felt like healing itself.

Second ICU Stay

Six weeks into recovery, I was deemed stable enough for surgery to remove the kidney stone and replace the stent. Hours later, my childhood friend noticed something was wrong. I was deteriorating—again.

Back to the ICU.

I had hypotension, high lactate and creatinine, and an elevated white cell count—sepsis, again. Cultures later confirmed Pseudomonas in my blood and Serratia in my urine. All my progress vanished. I couldn't even lift a spoon.

Depressed and Discouraged

Emotionally, this was my lowest point. I was exhausted and disheartened. After enduring three diagnostic tests that required me to lie still for an hour each, I was completely depleted.

The next morning, I saw a dry-erase board at the foot of my bed. It read:

"Goal: Ambulate." I couldn't even sit up.

Twice I tried. Twice I failed. Then I saw it—a photo taped to the grab bar: all nine of our grandchildren, smiling from a couch.

I remembered what I was fighting for. On the third try, I sat up. Then, with help, I stood. I cried—not from pain, but from hope.

One of our daughters-in-law had surrounded my space with family photos and voice messages. Those acts of love grounded me. I wasn't alone.

The Cost of Connection in a Pandemic

During my ICU stay, COVID-19 restrictions allowed only two designated visitors—one at a time, on alternating days. My husband, already drained, wasn't comfortable driving alone to the city. Thankfully, loving friends and family stepped up to drive him.

I knew I'd survive. But watching what this did to him—physically, emotionally, spiritually—was heartbreaking. Sometimes, I think our loved ones suffer more than we do. My prayers weren't for myself. They were for him.

Transitioning Again

After six days, I left the ICU. Some doctors wanted me transferred back to the original hospital for rehab, but I chose to stay where I was, to build strength until a proper rehab bed became available. From September 18–28, I slowly worked on regaining mobility while wounds and scarring continued to heal.

One bright spot was the arrival of second-year nursing students who rotated through each Thursday. They listened, wide-eyed, as I shared my story. I hoped I offered them a lesson in resilience—and the importance of listening to patients.

A Healing Bond in Rehab

On September 28, I was transferred to an inpatient rehab facility for a 19-day stay—an emotionally rich chapter in my recovery. There, I met the most incredible roommate. From our first conversation, we connected. We shared our stories, our tears, and our laughter. I believe we were the answer to each other's prayers.

We kept in touch after discharge, but heartbreakingly, she passed away a few months later from cancer. I still cry thinking of her. But I remain grateful for the bond we formed. She was a light in a dark time.

Coming Home to a Stranger's Life

I came home on October 17, 2020. My sister brought me. I slept in my own bed—though I didn't remember which room had been mine before. The house was familiar but felt different. My life had changed.

Summer had passed. Fall was underway. I wouldn't be hopping on the lawnmower anytime soon.

I now needed a walker, a shower chair, a bedrail, and grab bars. Occupational and physical therapists visited during the first month, helping me rebuild strength and confidence.

I encouraged my husband to resume his own routine. When I'm unwell, I don't want to be hovered over. I need space to find my footing on my terms.

Friends from church stocked our freezer with meals, though my appetite remained low for months. Even the hallway was a challenge to navigate. There were countless appointments—wound care, urology, physiatry, plastic surgery, and more.

My voice was barely audible. I relied on gestures and charades to communicate. It wasn't easy, but we made it work. I never had speech-language pathology, but I've booked a long-awaited appointment at a vocal clinic for August 2025. I'm finally ready to see what voice improvements may still be possible.

Endings and Beginnings

It took time to grasp all I had survived—septic shock, organ failure, emergency surgery. I spent 54 days across four hospitals and 19 more in rehab. I came home with wounds—some visible, some hidden—and a changed body and mind.

In November 2020, I had two more procedures: stent removal and fingertip amputation. Each brought new layers of healing.

I lost more than weight and muscle. I lost my voice, my stamina, and the energy that once fueled a life of service. I still grieve that loss—not being able to give as I once did.

But alongside the grief came growth. I gained clarity, resilience, and a deeper understanding of how to live with limits and still find meaning. Grief and gratitude can coexist. And they do, if we let them.

One Day at a Time

Recovery hasn't been linear. It's two steps forward, one back. Some days I feel strong. Others, fragile. But every day, I keep going.

My Occupational therapist encouraged me to contact our local Brain Injury Association. I was still experiencing memory lapses, trouble concentrating, and difficulty finding words. That connection became a turning point.

I also joined Sepsis Alliance Peer Support Conversations online. There, for the first time, I didn't have to explain. Other survivors already knew. That shared understanding gave me validation, comfort, and strength.

But I shouldn't have had to find those supports on my own. No one prepared me for what to expect post-sepsis. There were no clear roadmaps, no coordinated follow-ups, very little acknowledgment of the trauma I'd just endured, and even less on the Post-Sepsis Syndrome symptoms I was experiencing. There is a serious lack of resources for sepsis survivors—and it is nearly impossible to advocate for yourself when you are at your most vulnerable.

There have been moments of renewed hope. In late 2023, an ENT surgeon performed a delicate throat procedure that restored most of my voice. A plastic surgeon helped improve the function in my left hand. These weren't just medical wins—they were gifts of connection, independence, and expression.

I'm still adapting—building a life around this new reality. I find joy in small victories, such as remembering passwords, getting more than 5 hours of sleep, and having mornings with less exhaustion and pain. I carry scars, fatigue, and questions. But also, purpose and perspective.

Sepsis didn't just interrupt my life. It reshaped it. And in that reshaping, I've discovered a new kind of strength. I may never return to the life I had before. But that life no longer defines me.

This one does.

My Advice to New Survivors

I would want the survivor to realize that they are, or were, not the only victim of their sepsis experience. I wish that I had been more sensitive to my loved ones who were held hostage by what I went through. Actually, 5 years out, and they are still on the roller coaster ride with me.

At least it has slowed down, and the dips and turns aren't so sharp as before.

I became self-centred due to the attention I received in the hospital and within our community. Pre-sepsis, I was the one serving others in need. Post-sepsis, people were focused on me and my needs. I imagine that you are saying that I'm being too hard on myself right now. I regret that I couldn't relate to my husband's PTSD (finding me and seeing me on life support); my sister's fear/anxiety every time my husband's name and number show up on her Caller ID; and I could go on.

I would tell a survivor to look into the eyes of their caregivers and realize that they are victims of sepsis, too.

Linda Hart, Canada

My name is Linda, and I am a sepsis, Strep A, and an anaphylactic shock survivor. I am a "warrior" who fought a battle in my body without warning.

My journey began in May of 2018. I had an ovarian cyst removed with a recommended total hysterectomy. A few days after being discharged, I began to bleed from the incision, my blood pressure dropped, and I started going into shock. My husband called for an ambulance, and after being rushed to the hospital, we found out that I had an infection and went into septic shock.

I was given peptazole, an antibiotic to which my body had an allergic reaction. When a culture was taken to help diagnose my infection, the results came back as Strep A. This "perfect storm" affected the rest of my life and my family's life forever as we knew it.

Many times, sensitive decisions, surgeries, prayers, surgeons, nurses, plus a 7-month stay in the hospital began my journey to recovery. My memory of what happened is a blur. I only know what family and professionals have told me. Sepsis is life-altering, robbing people of choice and memory of time. It happens so quickly and takes so much.

In my scenario, I lost my bowels, part of my stomach, sensation in my tongue, my hands, and my legs below the knees. I am now a quad amputee with an ostomy.

Most of all, sepsis stole my hopes and dreams of my previous life. I struggled, but with great determination, I worked very hard to get to where I am today. I have an awesome support team encouraging me to move forward and live my best life. My husband Ken is my rock. He has been by my side through every hurdle and victory, while my family and friends send me strength and prayers to heal and flourish.

Many blessings have come my way during my journey. I have two perfect grandsons. Jase, whose name means "healer," has given me the strength I needed to work hard. He calls me Nana, showing empathy and acceptance of all my challenges. My second grandson, baby Bryce, has a name that means "strength." They are the true meaning of love and acceptance. They bring me so much joy.

I used to work at a daycare before my surgery, where I taught children about life lessons and how everyone has a story about what happens to them in their lives. Some people have happy times, while others have sad times. I am truly learning about life lessons and how to be humble and appreciate the good in people.

I try to smile and laugh every day, and usually, I receive a smile in return.

Life is good!

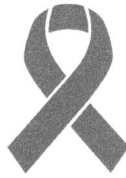

CHAPTER SEVEN

BRIDGING THE GAP: PATIENTS COLLABORATING WITH DOCTORS

There is a gap—a disconnect—between what we, as patients, know about our bodies and what our doctors see in a moment of crisis. That gap can be dangerous. But it can also be bridged.

I've learned, sometimes the hard way, that doctors are not the enemy. Most of them genuinely want to help. But they're human. They're under pressure, overloaded, and often walking into your hospital room with only a snapshot of your story. That's why your voice matters. Or, when you don't have a voice, having someone to speak up for you can be the difference between surviving and slipping through the cracks.

When You Can't Speak, You Need Someone Who Will

It is so important to have an advocate who can speak on your behalf in the beginning, because more often than not, you are too weak, too confused, or simply too out of it to advocate for yourself.

Three weeks ago, I was hospitalized again, this time with pancreatitis and an ileus. My port was also swollen and sore, and I had a gnawing suspicion that another sepsis infection was brewing. I told my husband we had to go to the ER.

By the time we got there, my abdomen was severely distended, the pain was through the roof, and I was vomiting. I couldn't even tell you when they called me back because the confusion had already started to settle in. My mind was slipping. I didn't recognize who was in the room. I didn't know when my husband left or when my daughters arrived. I was so lethargic and altered that the staff thought I might be having a stroke. They even did a CT scan of my head to be sure.

Meanwhile, my lab work was rolling in. My white blood cell count was 12.2—above the normal range—and a possible red flag for infection. But the doctor was about to dismiss it.

That's when my oldest daughter, who's a registered nurse, stepped in. She *knew* the signs of sepsis. She knew *me*. She showed the doctor pictures of my port and insisted—*insisted*—that he take it seriously. And thank God she did. He started me on Zosyn, a broad-spectrum antibiotic, right then and there. Within 30 minutes, the fog lifted. I could think again. I could recognize my daughters. I could express myself.

Turns out, my blood cultures were negative. No sepsis this time, thankfully. But I did have acute cellulitis in the area around my port. That infection, combined with the pancreatitis, was more than enough to derail my brain. And if my daughter hadn't spoken up, who knows how long I would have suffered in that state?

When You Can Speak, You Must

Once the confusion lifts and you're lucid enough to understand what's happening, it becomes *your* job to speak up. Communicate with your doctors and nurses clearly and directly, but always respectfully.

They're not mind-readers. And they don't know your history. Hospitals don't work the way they used to. Gone are the days when your regular doctor would follow your case while you were admitted. Now, it's hospitalists—doctors who are assigned to your care during your stay. They've never met you before. Often, they're too busy to comb through your records.

That's why you have to bring your history to *them*. You're not there to dictate. You are *part* of a team. But it's a team, and your voice matters.

Know Your Rights (and Use Them Wisely)

You do have rights. Important ones.

- You have the right to *refuse* care.
- You have the right to *fire* a doctor who you feel is not acting in your best interest.
- You have the right to *transfer* to another hospital if you are medically stable.
- You even have the right to *leave* AMA—against medical advice—if that's what you choose.

But I urge you to use those rights with wisdom. Doctors are human, just like you and me. They put their pants on one leg at a time. They have families. They get tired. They care deeply, even if they don't always show it. And just like any other relationship in your life, your connection with your doctor should be based on mutual respect. You'll accomplish so much more if you approach them as a partner rather than an opponent.

When All Else Fails—Call in Reinforcements

If you ever feel like you're at an impasse—if you're not being heard, if your care feels off, if something doesn't sit right with you—don't give up. Every hospital has patient advocates on staff. Their job is to help you and your medical team find common ground. Use them. That's what they're there for.

When You Know Your Body Better Than Anyone

There are times in your life—especially after surviving something like sepsis multiple times—when *you* become the expert on your own body.

In 2002, I had a gastric bypass with BPD—biliopancreatic diversion with duodenal switch. It's a complex surgery that's not commonly performed in the Midwest anymore. And because of that, many of the doctors and radiologists I encounter aren't familiar with my anatomy. That leads to misdiagnoses—*a lot* of them.

Luckily, my general surgeon, Dr. Opie, has performed every single one of my surgeries since that bypass. When he's available and at the hospital, he takes the time to educate the physicians around him. But if he's off, or on vacation, or not the one assigned to me, then it falls on *me* to fill in the gaps.

I have to speak up. I have to explain what's been done to my body. And so far, thankfully, the doctors have been receptive. Once they realize I'm not guessing, they listen. They proceed with caution. They pause before making assumptions.

But it's not just the surgery they need to know about.

I've had sepsis *thirteen times*. I've been in septic shock *twice*. That's not something they're going to find in a quick chart glance—especially now that a large university system has bought out my hospital. The electronic medical records system has changed, making many of my older records less accessible.

That lack of access to my history hinders continuity of care in an honestly scary way.

So again—it's on me to bring it up. I shouldn't *have* to. But I do. And so might you.

When They Don't Listen (And You Know Something's Wrong)

Whether it's your first time being sick or your tenth, it doesn't matter. You're not in that hospital bed or that ER chair for fun. You're there because you *feel like something's wrong.* Sometimes, when it's sepsis, it feels like you're going to die.

So when a medical professional dismisses that—when they tell you they're sending you home—it's enough to make your blood run cold.

You read a story in Chapter Six about Norma, who was sent home when she *should* have been admitted. And it changed her life forever. She still carries both the mental and physical scars of that decision. If she had been admitted, the outcome might have been very different. She might have been spared so much pain.

If your gut is screaming that going home is the wrong decision, you—or someone who loves you—needs to advocate strongly for a 23-hour observation stay. Hospitals can do that without officially admitting you. It gives the doctor time to evaluate your condition more thoroughly, and it gives you a chance to be monitored.

And if that still doesn't work? Go to another hospital.

Seriously. I know that sounds extreme, but this is *your life*. If one ER sends you home and you know something's still terribly wrong, find another one that might take it more seriously. Don't let pride or fear of "bothering" someone keep you from getting the help you need.

If all else fails—and I mean *all else*—call your regular doctor, even if it's after hours. Ask them to intervene. But please, only use this option as a last resort. It's not meant to be the first step. Let your primary doctor rest unless the situation truly demands it.

When You're Dismissed

We previously visited this story, but it's worth mentioning again as it serves as an excellent reminder of why patient advocacy is non-negotiable.

My husband was out of town, and I started running a fever. In my world, that's never just a fever—it's a warning siren. Within 30 minutes, my temperature hit 102°. I knew I had to act fast. I called my grandson to come stay with the dogs, grabbed my go-bag—which I always keep packed for the hospital—and drove myself to the ER.

Once I got there, of course, my fever had subsided. That happens sometimes. It doesn't mean I'm in the clear, but it can fool people who aren't familiar with my past experiences. And unfortunately, that night, it did.

The nurse barely listened to me. She didn't seem concerned. And because she brushed it off, the doctor followed her lead. He entered the room with a dismissive tone and showed no genuine curiosity. He wasn't planning to do *anything*—no labs, no physical exam, not even listening to my whole history. They were just going to send me home.

That had *never* happened to me before.

Usually, the minute I mention my multiple episodes of sepsis, two of septic shock—ears perk up. Questions follow. Tests are ordered. But not that night.

I protested. I stayed calm, but I didn't back down. And you know what he said?

"What is it you want me to do?"

Can you imagine? I looked him in the eye and said, "At the very least, I want lab work and blood cultures done. Then I'll be happy to go home."

He agreed—grudgingly—but he never once laid a hand on me. No physical exam. Not even a stethoscope to the chest.

As a healthcare professional myself, I was disgusted. I later filed a formal hospital complaint. They never followed up with me—not even to ask for details. That's shameful, and honestly, it tarnishes the hospital's reputation. What if the next patient doesn't know how to advocate? What if they go home and don't make it?

That night was the *exception*, not the rule. I want to be clear about that. Every other time I've gone to the ER for sepsis or something else, I've been treated with compassion and seriousness.

The Power of True Collaboration

Even with the occasional setback, I have to say: more often than not, I've had wonderful experiences with ER doctors—especially when I'm facing sepsis.

Sepsis is a monster. It doesn't wait. It doesn't give you a chance to ease into the crisis. One minute you're okay, and the next you're crashing. Collaboration between the patient and the doctor is so vital. There's no time for egos or assumptions.

I've been fortunate. In many of my admissions, the ER physicians have stopped what they were doing to really *listen* to me. I'll start telling my story—what I've been through, what symptoms are appearing, what my gut is telling me—and that's when I see it: their entire posture changes. They start to look into my history. They connect the dots. And then we work *together*.

Maybe it's because I'm a nurse. Perhaps it's because I am confident in my conversations. I don't know. But I do know this: those partnerships have saved my life over and over again.

There's something powerful about being seen by your doctor as an equal—someone who understands their body, who knows the signs, and who brings valuable insight to the table. I've found that the more I educate myself about my own health—and the clearer I am about what I expect from my care—the more I'm respected and trusted.

Over time, the relationships I've built with my health-care providers—pulmonologists, infectious disease doctors, occupational and physical therapists, interventional radiologists—have evolved. We've developed genuine relationships. They have become partners in my care who walk alongside me through the storm, and together, we've built care plans based on mutual respect and shared goals.

That trust didn't happen overnight. It took time. But it started with me learning to speak up and stay open, even when I was scared or exhausted. It grew from showing that I respected their expertise while still standing firmly.

To any survivor reading this who feels unsure or intimidated about speaking up: I've been there. I know what it's like to question if you're being "too much" or fear that you're stepping on toes.

You are not just a patient. You are a partner in your care.

Whether you're too weak to talk and need someone to advocate for you, or you're strong enough to tell your story clearly, your role in your healthcare is necessary. And when you collaborate with your providers from a place of mutual respect, incredible things can happen.

I've survived sepsis thirteen times. I've had good doctors, and I've had bad nights. But the thread running through it all—the thing that's kept me alive—is this: I've learned how to be heard.

And so can you.

You are your own best advocate. Never forget that.

KEY TAKEAWAYS

➢ Having a trusted advocate when you're too weak or confused to speak up can be the difference between getting life-saving care or slipping through the cracks.

➢ Once you're able, it's essential to clearly and respectfully communicate your history, symptoms, and concerns—doctors are not mind-readers, and your voice matters.

➢ You have legal rights as a patient, but using them wisely and with mutual respect for your providers often leads to the best outcomes.

➢ If something feels off and you're not being heard, don't give up—use hospital advocates, ask for observation status, or even seek care elsewhere.

➢ Building strong relationships with your healthcare team takes time, but when you speak with knowledge and respect, you earn trust—and that trust can save your life.

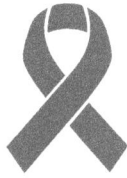

CHAPTER EIGHT

BUILDING A COMMUNITY OF SEPSIS ADVOCATES

Sepsis can leave you reeling physically, emotionally, and mentally. You survive it, yes. But then what? Many survivors are left to navigate the aftermath alone, without a clear map or a community to lean on. Connection saves lives. Survivors need each other. We need to be heard, seen, and understood. And we need to use what we've lived through to reach back and help the next person up.

I didn't start out thinking I was going to be an advocate. But there was a point when I knew I had to be.

Several years after my first sepsis episode, I reached out to the hospital where I'd worked as a nurse. I contacted their sepsis team, hoping to contribute in some way, especially since I had insider experience both as a healthcare professional and a patient. I thought surely they'd want input from someone who'd been through it. But they weren't interested. They weren't focused on patient education at all. That interaction left me frustrated and disappointed. It felt like a door slammed shut.

So I turned to the people who *did* want to talk: other survivors. My work didn't begin with some grand plan. It started organically. In the early days, I just offered support—a shoulder to cry on. I found myself reaching out to people who were struggling, and I let them know I was there for them, whenever they needed someone. I joined Facebook groups, offering encouragement and a listening ear to those just beginning their recovery. That's where the spark really started. I saw how powerful it was to connect with others who understood.

When Sepsis Alliance started developing its virtual support groups, something nudged me to step forward. They were offering facilitator training, and I decided to go for it. Mind you, this wasn't during an easy time in my life.

I was recovering from major back surgery at the time. One of my sepsis infections had led to osteomyelitis, discitis, and burst fractures of my T9 and T10 vertebrae, which had trapped my spinal cord. I had rods and pins placed from T7 to T12. I couldn't even sit comfortably for long periods. But I pushed through.

I'll never forget that first test support group. It lasted 90 minutes, and I was physically uncomfortable the whole time, but I finished it. And when it was over, I felt something I hadn't felt in a long time: *good*. It was uplifting. Gratifying. Like I had finally found something meaningful in the mess of what I'd been through.

That first group ignited something in me, and I've never looked back. Over the past three years, I think I've only missed one session, and that was for an important doctor's appointment. The group meets every other Thursday afternoon, and it's one of the highlights of my life.

From there, the connections just kept growing. I started a second group—a ladies' coffee group for sepsis survivors. We meet on Zoom. Our conversations aren't always about sepsis, but the shared experience of surviving it ties us together in a way that's hard to describe. We laugh, we cry, we vent. We talk about life after trauma, about joy, grief, hope, and everything in between. Some of the relationships I've built in that group are deep and lasting. These women have become my sisters in survival.

The Emotional Shift to Advocacy

When I first became an advocate, something inside me changed. After retiring from nursing—something I had loved doing for years—I felt insignificant. The part of me that gave and nurtured and helped people had been stripped away. Sepsis had taken so much from me physically, but the emotional weight of losing my career and sense of purpose was just as heavy.

But when I stepped into that first support group as a facilitator, I felt uplifted. I felt *hope* for my future again. For the first time in a long time, I felt like I had a purpose—to help others through something I deeply understood. That's where my healing truly began.

Facilitating support groups has helped me grow in ways I didn't expect. I get to work with people who are newly post-sepsis. I can look them in the eye—whether in person or on Zoom—and say, "You're not alone." I help validate their feelings, confusion, grief, and fears. I remind them that others have walked this path before them and are here to help pave the way forward.

We Can't Do It Alone

As survivors, we do everything we can to be there for one another. We show up. We listen. We share our stories. But real change also has to come from the very system that treated us—and too often, released us without preparing us for what came next.

Hospitals and healthcare providers have a vital role to play in helping us survive sepsis *and* in helping us live *afterward*. So if I had just five minutes to speak directly to those in charge—those who can make the system better for the next survivor—here's exactly what I'd say.

To Hospital Administrators:

Please—set up programs to educate and support sepsis survivors and their families. Most people leave the hospital with no idea what sepsis even is, let alone what to expect when they get home. That's not acceptable.

Give them written materials they can refer back to later. Don't assume they'll remember what you say while they're still foggy or traumatized. Provide community resources they can turn to—brain injury support groups, physical therapy, counseling, and more.

Create support groups for:

- Survivors
- Caregivers
- People who've lost loved ones to sepsis

And don't stop there. Launch community education campaigns. Help the public understand what signs and symptoms to watch out for before it's too late.

To Doctors and Nurses:

Tell your patients they've had sepsis or septic shock. You'd be shocked at how many don't even know. Then explain what that means. Talk to them about Post-Sepsis Syndrome and PTSD. About the emotional roller coaster they might face. Let them know what symptoms to expect after discharge and when those symptoms might be a red flag.

Validate their fears. Don't brush them off. Don't rush out of the room.

Answer their questions. And if you don't know the answer,

say so—and then go find it. That one act can mean the world to someone who feels lost in their own body.

Let patients know that their feelings are normal. That they're not crazy, and what they're going through is part of the healing process. Be available to listen. Even if you can't fix it, just listen.

And lastly, educate your staff. Every member of the care team should be aligned because continuity of care matters. Survivors need to feel like they're supported by a united front, not like they're being passed from one disconnected hand to another.

Healing Through Helping

Healing really began for me once I started being there for others. There's just something powerful about watching someone appear in a group for the first time—depressed, anxious, overwhelmed—and then watching the light return to their face when they realize they're not alone. What they're feeling is real, and there's a whole group of people who *get it* because we've lived it.

I've had people say to me, "You've had *thirteen* episodes of sepsis? Aren't you scared to death?" And my answer is honest: "Yes. Of course, I'm afraid of getting it again. But now I know what to look for. And at the first sign, I go straight to the ER."

When I say that, I see the fear melt off their face. That moment is why I keep going.

Do I ever feel discouraged? Absolutely.

It's heartbreaking when someone reaches out to me in desperation—asking for help—and then disappears before we can connect again. I always hope that when they're truly ready, they reach out to *someone*, even if it's not me or our group. I hope they find the help they need and the courage to take that next step.

And it's just as disheartening when I try to advocate to doctors—sharing information about Post-Sepsis Syndrome—and their eyes glaze over. Or they politely take the literature I hand them and likely toss it in the trash. I know they're busy. I get it. But even *one act* of listening could change everything for a patient who feels lost and scared.

That's why I'm so grateful for my primary care physician, Dr. Newkirk. He listens. He treats me like a partner in my own care. That kind of relationship is rare, and I cherish it.

You Don't Have to Be Loud to Be an Advocate

If you're reading this and thinking, *I'm not sure I could ever be an advocate,* I want to tell you—yes, you can. Advocacy doesn't have to mean standing on a stage or leading a group. It starts with something simple: *telling your story.*

You can start small. Share what you went through with a friend. Post a little bit about your journey on social media. You'd be amazed at how many people will respond.

Some will say, "I went through something similar." Others

will say, "My dad died from sepsis. I never even knew what it was until now." Those connections are where advocacy begins.

There is healing in community. There is power in speaking up. And there is a deep, soul-restoring purpose in being a light for someone else who's just now stepping out of the dark.

Be that light.

Tell your story.

And know that you're not just surviving—you're helping the rest of us survive too.

KEY TAKEAWAYS

➢ Advocacy doesn't have to be loud or formal—it begins with sharing your story and showing up for others who feel alone.

➢ True healing often starts when survivors find purpose in helping others navigate post-sepsis life.

➢ Survivors need support groups, community, and validation, especially from those who've lived through it and from compassionate medical professionals.

➢ Hospitals and healthcare providers must do more to educate patients and offer resources that extend beyond discharge.

➢ Even the smallest acts of connection—listening, validating, and sharing—can transform fear into hope for someone struggling to heal.

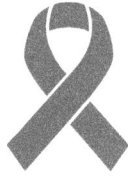

CHAPTER NINE

THE WAY FORWARD: HOPE, HEALING, AND ADVOCACY

Looking back across all thirteen times I survived sepsis, I can tell you this: it changed me. At my core, I am not the same person I was before.

But I'm stronger now. I don't sweat the small stuff anymore. I don't waste energy worrying about things that don't matter. I appreciate life more deeply. I appreciate my family and friends in a way I never did before. When you've come close to death that many times, you see everything differently. You stop taking things—or people—for granted.

There are days I grieve for the old me. I miss feeling good. I miss having energy. I miss getting to eat normally, like everyone else. I miss going out whenever I want, being with friends, laughing over dinner without worrying about my body giving out.

I miss being a nurse. I miss taking care of people. That was such a huge part of who I was. I miss being the matriarch of my family—the one who held everything and everyone together.

But even with the extensive health problems I now live with, I refuse to play the victim. I will not sit in that role. I don't want to be seen as "the patient." In my mind, I'm just a regular person, living life day by day like anyone else.

Even though I can't work as a nurse anymore, I still get to care for people—just in a different way now. I love answering medical questions from other sepsis survivors. I don't give medical advice, but I help people understand their journey better. I help them make sense of what they've been through. It's powerful, and it gives me purpose.

And yes, I wish I could travel the country, standing before big audiences, testifying before Congress, and making change on a national level. But I also know my physical limitations. So I do what I can, where I am. I spread the word. I tell the truth. I support survivors directly—one voice, one message, one person at a time.

Why I Still Have Hope

There's a lot that needs to change in how we treat and understand sepsis, but I do have hope. One of the most important developments is that we finally have an actual diagnosis code for Post- Sepsis Syndrome (PSS). That might sound small, but it's significant. Doctors can no longer ignore it or pretend it doesn't exist. I hope that with this code, more doctors will become open to learning about PSS. And when that happens, they'll be better equipped to help patients walk through their recovery journey. They'll be more likely to listen. More likely to explain what caused the sepsis. More likely to help patients know what to watch for next time. And they'll hopefully be more willing to run additional tests when something feels off— because sepsis survivors know when something isn't right.

I would love to see every hospital establish a sepsis team dedicated solely to supporting patients and caregivers through-out their hospital stay. That team could help educate people on what's happening, advocate for next steps, and start mapping out a solid road to recovery before the patient ever goes home.

I want to see hospitals create their own support groups—for survivors, for caregivers, and even for people who've lost some-one to sepsis. Everyone affected needs a space where they can feel heard, seen, and supported.

There's something else that gives me hope, and that's AI— Artificial Intelligence. I know there's a lot of fear around AI in healthcare, but when it comes to sepsis, I'm excited about it. Because sepsis moves fast, catching it early is the difference between life and death.

AI has the power to spot things that even the best doctors and nurses might miss. It can monitor vital signs, lab results, and medical records all at once—something no single person can realistically do. It can recognize subtle changes or patterns and send an alert before things spiral, resulting in faster diagnosis, faster treatment, and better odds of survival.

AI doesn't replace the care team. But it can support them. It can act like an early warning system—an extra set of eyes that never sleeps. And in the world of sepsis, this can save lives and reduce long-term complications. That's the kind of progress I want to see more of.

To Every Survivor: You Are Not Broken

If you're reading this and you're still in the dark, afraid, or feeling broken—I want you to know something:

There is life after sepsis.

It might not be the life you imagined. It might not be like it was before sepsis. But that doesn't mean it can't still be full. It can be fulfilling. It can even be better than it was before. Surviving sepsis gives you a new perspective. It strips away the stuff that doesn't matter and shows you what's really important.

I live with a lot of invisible disabilities: severe fatigue, stage 3b kidney failure from the toxic antibiotics and vasopressors (medications used to raise blood pressure), chronic anemia, endocrine disorders such as hyperparathyroidism and hypothyroidism, feeling cold all of the time, difficulties regulating temperature extremes (both heat and cold), malnutrition, spinal deformities, a compromised immune system, chronic aches and pains, cognitive deficiencies such as brain fog, memory problems, difficulty with attention and concentration, difficulty finding words, sleep disturbances, swelling in extremities, peripheral neuropathy, and more. These are the lasting effects of sepsis. However, I also know that things could have turned out much worse.

First and foremost, I survived.

I have the love and support of my family. I have my best friend—my twin sister from another mother—by my side. And even though I lost some friends who couldn't handle my illness, I've gained even more who understand and lift me up. People like Myrna, Norma, Gail, Anika, Jen, Penny, Don, Darrell, Andrew, Van, Steven—and many others.

My life is full.

And yours can be too. Don't give up. Don't hide. You are not broken. You are still here. That means something.

To the Caregivers: Please Don't Forget Yourself

For the families and caregivers out there, especially the ones walking through this journey with a loved one, I see you. I am you. I take care of my mother, who lives with us and has vascular dementia, so I know firsthand how heavy that responsibility can feel.

Take care of yourself. You are no good to anyone if you are run down physically or emotionally. I know it feels selfish sometimes, but it's not. It's necessary. Eat healthy. Move your body. Work off your frustrations—don't let them sit inside you.

Find support. Don't try to do this alone. There are Facebook groups for caregivers of sepsis survivors. There's Sepsis Alliance Connect's Caregiver Support Group on Zoom (visit_sepsisconnect.org). Seek out respite care, even if it's just for an afternoon. Go run errands. Get a massage. Take a nap. Refill your cup.

A Message to Medical Professionals: We Need You

To the healthcare professionals who want to do better—thank you. We need more of you. And here's what I want you to know.

There's an incredible resource out there just for you: the Sepsis Alliance Institute. It's built specifically for medical professionals. You'll find education, tools, webinars (many with CEUs), and a community of peers who are passionate about improving sepsis care. Get involved. Join webinars with your coworkers. Learn together.

I once participated in a panel as a sepsis survivor alongside several others. We shared our stories with healthcare professionals, answered questions, and had real, honest conversations about what it was like—both in the hospital and after we went home. That panel was one of the most well-received experiences I've ever been a part of. And it showed me that you want to understand. You want to help.

So don't go it alone. Use the tools. Make the time. Connect with your peers. This is a one-stop shop that can help you care better—and help survivors like me feel seen, heard, and truly supported.

My Hope. My Legacy.

If I could leave behind just one thing with all this advocacy, I hope it's this:

That every sepsis survivor knows that their voice matters. That their experience is real. That their journey doesn't end when they're discharged from the hospital.

There is life after sepsis. It's different, yes. It's hard. It's complicated. But it's still life. And it can still be meaningful, beautiful, and full of connection.

For healthcare providers, my hope is just as clear: Please listen to us. Take us seriously. Validate what we're going through—even when it doesn't show up on a chart. We don't need false reassurance. We need the truth. Tell us that we have sepsis. We often don't hear that diagnosis until after discharge. We need to know that the long road of recovery might stretch on for years, even a lifetime, but that we won't be walking it alone.

That's the legacy I want to leave behind. A world where survivors are empowered. A system where care continues beyond the crisis. And a conversation that includes all of us—patients, caregivers, and medical professionals—working together to build something better.

Because surviving sepsis isn't the end of the story, it's the beginning of a whole new chapter.

And we're writing it together.

KEY TAKEAWAYS

➤ Surviving sepsis changes you, but it doesn't diminish your worth—there is still a full and meaningful life ahead.

➤ Even when you can't return to who you were before, you can still live with purpose, helping others in new and powerful ways.

➤ Progress is being made from the recognition of Post-Sepsis Syndrome to the promise of AI in early detection, which gives real hope.

➤ Caregivers matter too, and their health, rest, and support are just as essential as the survivor's recovery.

➤ Advocacy starts with one voice at a time—every survivor, caregiver, and medical professional has the power to make a difference.

EPILOGUE

"Don't let fear get in the way of your destiny."
– Author unknown

First and foremost, congratulations on beating sepsis. By reading my book, you've shown that you are sick and tired of being sick and tired. That takes courage. As I close this chapter of my story, I do so with deep gratitude—for life, for the people who have carried me through, and for the chance to share my journey with you. Surviving sepsis not once, but thirteen times, has taught me that resilience is not about avoiding hardship, but about finding the strength to rise after each fall.

I know that life after sepsis is not the same. Our bodies may be altered, and our paths forever changed. But we are still here—still living, still capable of joy, still valuable. If you take one message from my story, let it be this: you are not alone. Whether you are a survivor, a caregiver, or someone just beginning to understand sepsis, know that there is a community ready to support and uplift you.

Survival alone is not enough. If you delay dealing with your recovery—physically or emotionally—the weight of sepsis can linger, holding you back from living fully. Unspoken fears may grow stronger, your body may struggle longer, and hope may feel further away. However, taking even small steps toward recovery—such as seeking support, caring for your health, and giving yourself grace—can make all the difference. You've already proven your strength in survival; now give yourself the chance to heal.

I hope that these pages have given you encouragement, understanding, and the courage to share your own story. Together, by raising awareness and standing together, we can ensure that no one faces sepsis or its aftermath in silence.

Here's a simple way to begin:

1. **Share Your Story** – Your experience has power. Whether through writing, speaking, or posting on social media, sharing what you've been through raises awareness and helps others feel less alone.

2. **Connect with Organization**s – Join groups such as Sepsis Alliance or local health advocacy organizations. They offer resources, training, and opportunities to get involved in spreading awareness and supporting survivors.

3. **Start Small** – Advocacy doesn't have to be overwhelming. Begin with small actions, such as posting on World Sepsis Day, speaking with your local hospital, or joining a support group—and let your efforts grow over time.

You've survived something that tried to take everything from you. Don't let fear hold you back from living the life you were meant to live. Your destiny is still unfolding, and you have the power to shape it.

ADDENDUM

As this book is going to press, I was admitted to the hospital on Monday, November 24, 2025, with my 14th episode of sepsis. This infection began as cellulitis in my right lower extremity, which was edematous, and progressed when bacteria migrated to my portacath. I spent Thanksgiving in the hospital and was finally discharged Saturday, November 29, 2025.

ABOUT SANDRA KLEIER

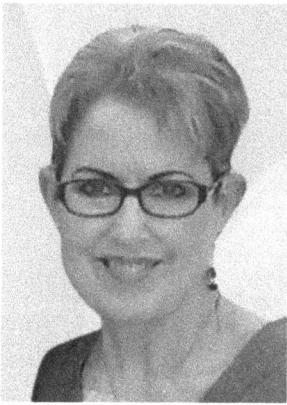

Sandra Kleier is an RN of 34 years, now medically retired post-sepsis. She and her husband, Ron, live on a 16-acre farm in rural Kansas with their three dogs and 14 cats. She's a caregiver for her live-in mother with vascular dementia.

Sandra serves as Treasurer on her local Township board and Treasurer for the Wellsville High School Class of 1981 Scholarship Committee. She volunteers for Sepsis Alliance Connect by facilitating a Sepsis Support Group for Sepsis Survivors via Zoom. Sandra has participated in several panels for webinars for sepsis survivors and healthcare professionals through Sepsis Alliance.

In her spare time, she enjoys spending time with her six children and 13 grandchildren. She also enjoys reading, doing crafts, gardening, and relaxing under a shade tree in the hammock chairs.

www.ingramcontent.com/pod-product-compliance
Lightning Source LLC
Chambersburg PA
CBHW060905280326
41934CB00007B/1190